The
DICTIONARY
OF
MEDICINE

The DICTIONARY OF MEDICINE

Galley Press

Galley Press

© Copyright Marshall Editions Limited 1986,
1989
170 Piccadilly, London W1V 9DD

Published in this edition 1989 by Galley Press,
an imprint of W H Smith Limited
Registered No. 237811 England
Trading as WHS Distributors, St John's House
East Street, Leicester, LE1 6NE

ISBN 0 86136 181 4

1 2 3 4 5 93 92 91 90 89

Printed in Italy by Gruppo Editoriale Fabbri S.p.A., Milan.

HOW TO USE THIS BOOK

This A to Z book is a vital reference work for anyone who needs rapid, full and up-to-date information on the many themes of modern medicine and medical practice. Its information-packed pages include the following:

- Descriptions of the diseases and disorders of the world, their symptoms and associated side effects.
- Conditions of the body, normal and abnormal.
- The parts of the body, their functions and the way they work.
- Equipment used by doctors and medical specialists and technicians.
- Diagnostic methods, tests, treatments and therapeutic techniques.
- Technicalities and technical terms.

In addition there are many brief biographies of major doctors and medical scientists past and present; information about health and fitness and on the way in which infections are contracted; and illustrations of key aspects of body anatomy and physiology.

It must be emphasized that despite the comprehensive coverage of medicine contained in this dictionary, it is not intended in any way as a means to self-diagnosis of diseases and disorders. No book can substitute for the personal knowledge and experience of a trained medical practitioner. For all that, the use of this volume may lead to a greater understanding of medical knowledge and practice, which may enable a person to describe more fully and accurately any signs or symptoms to his or her doctor when overtaken by ill health.

The use of the book for encyclopedic reading is made possible by the careful and consistent indication of cross-references. A word or phrase within an entry that appears in SMALL CAPITAL letters also has its own entry, under that word or phrase as its heading, at the appropriate point in the alphabet. The reader can thus, if wished, proceed from entry to entry by referring to new headings until a whole subject area is fully explored.

A

abdomen the large, lined body cavity that lies between the diaphragm and the pelvic floor. It contains a number of organs, including the LIVER and INTESTINES.

abortion the induced termination of PREGNANCY, generally sometime up to 20 weeks — in some areas, 28 weeks — after conception. Spontaneous termination is called a miscarriage.

abrasion a superficial wound caused by scraping the skin; blood may be drawn.

abreaction the psychiatric term for the emotional release following a patient's recollection of a previously repressed painful experience.

abscess a well-defined collection of PUS in a body tissue, often caused by BACTERIA.

accommodation an adjustment in the shape of the lens of the eye to enable it to focus an image of an object on the retina.

acetabulum the socket of the hip joint. It is the cup-shaped part made up of two pelvic bones — the ilium and the ischium — into which the head of the thighbone (femur) fits.

acetylcholine a chemical NEUROTRANS-MITTER secreted at some neural synapses when nerve impulses are to be passed on from one nerve ending to another.

ache a dull, usually continuous pain.

achilles tendon the strong fibrous band that joins the bone of the heel to the muscles at the back of the lower leg; it enables these muscles to lift the heel during walking or running.

acid a chemical compound that usually forms a salt and water when it reacts with a base, releasing hydrogen ions. There are a number of body acids, most significantly those that aid digestion in the stomach.

acidosis a condition in which the blood is more acidic than normal. There are many causes of acidosis, including disorders of the lungs and kidneys, which are responsible for maintaining normal acidity.

acne a skin complaint most commonly affecting teenagers, and manifested in pimples, particularly on the face and the upper parts of the body.

acquired immune deficiency syndrome the full name for the disease also called AIDS.

acromegaly a disorder in which the bones and tissues of the extremities — the nose, jaws, fingers and toes — become abnormally enlarged. It is caused by over-production of GROWTH HORMONE from the PITUITARY GLAND.

acromion process part of the shoulder blade or SCAPULA.

ACTH (adrenocorticotropic hormone) a hormone produced by the PITUITARY GLAND at the base of the brain. It stimulates the outer layer of the ADRENAL GLANDS above the kidneys to produce other hormones, and in a synthesized form may be administered to relieve symptoms of RHEUMATISM, MULTIPLE SCLEROSIS and ASTHMA.

actin a protein in the supporting structure of body cells. It associates with MYOSIN in muscular contraction.

acupuncture a method of treatment, originating in ancient China, in which long needles are inserted into the body at precise points to relieve pain, or to treat other conditions. In the West it is still considered an unorthodox treatment and commonly classified among types of ALTERNATIVE MEDICINE.

acute describes a condition that comes on suddenly and — following appropriate treatment — lasts a comparatively short time, as distinct from a CHRONIC condition.

addiction an uncontrollable physical or psychological dependence on a substance or a pattern of behavior — such as ALCOHOL or other drugs, or gambling.

Addison, Thomas (1793–1869) an English physician who was the first to recognize a disorder of the ADRENAL GLANDS, later named ADDISON'S DISEASE. It has been suggested that the science of endocrinology dates from his discovery.

Addison's disease an uncommon condition that occurs when the adrenal cortex (the outer layer of the ADRENAL GLAND above the kidney) fails to produce certain essential steroid HORMONES. The symptoms are weakness, loss of weight, low blood pressure and, in Caucasians, a darkening of the skin.

adenoids two small masses of lymphoid tissue located at the back of the nasal passage. They protect the respiratory system by capturing and destroying inhaled germs. If seriously infected they can be surgically removed. They are sometimes known as pharangyeal tonsils.

adenoma a benign (noncancerous) tumor either on a gland or forming a glandlike structure. A cancerous or malignant version is called an adenocarcinoma.

adenosine diphosphate *see* ADP.

adenosine monophosphate *see* AMP.

adenosine triphosphate *see* ATP.

adhesion is a band of fibrous scar tissue connecting two internal body surfaces which are not normally joined.

adipose means fatty, or containing fat. Adipose tissue stores fat in the body.

Adler, Alfred (1870–1937) an Austrian physician and psychiatrist who advanced the theory of the inferiority complex to explain psychopathic cases. He claimed that NEUROSIS arises from efforts to compensate for feelings of inferiority which resulted in overcompensation. Originally a follower of Sigmund FREUD, Adler later devised the school of thinking called individual psychology.

adolescence the time between PUBERTY and sexual maturity, when the activity of the sex glands causes physical and emotional changes.

ADP (adenosine diphosphate) a NUCLEOTIDE (a compound formed of phosphoric acid, a sugar and a base). The conversion of ATP (adenosine triphosphate) to ADP is accompanied by the release of energy which may be used for many different cellular functions within the human body.

adrenal gland an ENDOCRINE GLAND located above each kidney. It produces a range of hormones.

adrenaline another name for the hormone EPINEPHRINE.

adrenocorticotropic hormone *see* ACTH.

aerobic describes a process that depends on oxygen. Aerobic exercises, or aerobics, is a system of physical exercises designed to maintain fitness by speeding up the breathing, thus increasing oxygen usage and stimulating blood circulation.

Aesculapius the Roman name for the Greek god of medicine, ASKLEPIOS.

afterbirth the collection of tissues expelled from the WOMB after childbirth. It is made up of the PLACENTA and other membranes.

aging the process of growing old. Physical characteristics of aging include an increasingly stooped posture, wrinkling of the skin, stiffening of the joints, thinning of the hair, and lessening of muscle strength.

agoraphobia fear of open spaces.

AID the abbreviation for the process of ARTIFICIAL INSEMINATION in which sperm is provided by a donor.

AIDS (acquired immune deficiency syndrome) in its active form an extremely serious, presently incurable disease now known to be caused by one, or possibly two or three, specific viruses which attack and destroy the patient's IMMUNE SYSTEM. The result is the undefended invasion by other infective agents, leading sometimes to serious infections and malignant tumors. The virus is passed on in infected blood or in semen during sexual intercourse; the time span between infection and appearance of symptoms indicating the active form of infection is not known, although a period of six years has been suggested.

AIH the abbreviation for the process of ARTIFICIAL INSEMINATION in which sperm is provided by the recipient's husband.

air embolism a specific type of EMBOLISM caused by the presence of an air bubble in a blood vessel. Sufficiently large, one may block the blood flow.

albino describes an individual who has a hereditary condition (albinism) in which the skin, hair, and eyes lack the dark coloring matter (pigment) MELANIN.

albumin a PROTEIN that occurs in various forms in milk, in the white of egg and in the blood. Its function is to maintain the correct balance of water in the body and to transport hormones and other substances.

albuminuria also called proteinuria, the presence of the protein albumin in the urine. Undetectable except through tests, it is found in a number of kidney conditions, ranging from minor temporary disorders to chronic irreversible disease.

alcohol is the common name for ethyl alcohol, a colorless, flammable liquid produced by the fermentation of sugars, which in quantity has poisonous effects on the central nervous system and other organs. It can be used as an antiseptic, a painkiller, or for several other medicinal purposes, but is most commonly encountered in alcoholic drinks. Drunkenness is a mild form of alcohol poisoning.

alcoholism an ADDICTION to alcohol. Like many addictions, it is associated with psychological, physical and social symptoms, such as aggressiveness and the deterioration of intellectual processes.

aldosterone a steroid HORMONE produced by the outer layer of each ADRENAL GLAND. It regulates the level of mineral salts in the blood and helps to control blood volume.

alimentary canal another name for the digestive tract, the tube which runs from the mouth to the anus.

alkaloid any of a varied group of chemicals that contain nitrogen, and have an effect on human metabolism. Many — including caffeine, nicotine, cocaine, morphine and digitalis — are found in plants, and in quantity may be poisonous. Some are used as drugs.

allergen any substance that causes an ALLERGY.

allergy an abnormal sensitivity to any substance that does not adversely affect most people. The sensitivity causes an adverse physical reaction, which often takes the form of a RASH, but can also include symptoms such as sneezing or vomiting.

alopecia the medical term for BALDNESS.

alternative medicine the name given to a number of therapies that depart in principle and practice from orthodox and established medicine. Many prefer to treat the individual patient as a whole, by means of "HOLISTIC" methods. Alternative therapies that rely to a greater or lesser extent on physical manipulation include CHIROPRACTIC, OSTEOPATHY, reflexology, and the Alexander Technique. NATUROPATHY also includes some massage. Dietary remedies (including the administering of certain solutions and the drinking of liquids) are to be found in HOMEOPATHY, NATUROPATHY, herbalism, and hydrotherapy. ACUPUNCTURE involves the insertion of needles into the skin. Thought control methods include autogenic training and hypnotherapy.

altitude sickness, or mountain sickness a condition of stress that may occur at high altitudes, where atmospheric pressure is lower and there is less oxygen in the air. As a result, the red blood cells cannot take in enough oxygen, which at least initially causes the breathing rate to rise. Symptoms include shortness of breath, fatigue, headache and fainting.

alveolus one of the microscopic air sacs in the lungs where gas exchange occurs.

Alzheimer's disease formerly called presenile dementia, a condition in which the brain progressively degenerates before the onset of old age.

ameba any of a group of microscopic one-celled animals, some species of which can live in the human body. Amebae can infect the colon, causing amebic DYSENTERY, a diarrheal illness which is common in the tropics and is usually spread through contaminated drinking water; they can also cause abscesses, particularly in the liver.

amebiasis the condition of being infected with AMEBAE.

amebic dysentery a type of DYSENTERY caused by infection with AMEBAE.

amenorrhea the absence of menstruation in a woman. It is normal before MENARCHE and after the MENOPAUSE.

amino acid any one of twenty or more organic compounds that form the building blocks of PROTEINS. All contain nitrogen, oxygen, carbon and hydrogen, and most are synthesized by the body itself. "Essential" amino acids are the eight that the human body cannot itself synthesize and must regularly obtain from the diet in foods such as meat, milk or eggs.

ammonia a pungent, colorless, soluble gas that is a normal constituent of blood. An alkali, it is excreted in urine, in which it helps to neutralize acid.

amnesia a partial or total loss of long-term memory. Causes include disease or physical injury to the brain, DRUG

ADDICTION, ALCOHOLISM, and emotional disturbance.

amniocentesis   the removal of a sample of fluid from the amniotic sac (amnion) surrounding a fetus, to test for genetic abnormalities.

amnion   the inner membrane of the fluid-filled sac in which an unborn baby in the womb "floats".

AMP (adenosine monophosphate)   a NUCLEOTIDE (a compound formed of phosphoric acid, a sugar and a base) which is convertible to ADP and ATP. It plays an important part in biochemistry.

amputation   the cutting off of part of the body. Surgical amputation may be carried out in cases of untreatable disease or irreparable damage.

anabolic steroids   hormones, sometimes prescribed as supplementary DRUGS, which promote tissue growth.

anaerobic   living or active in the absence of free oxygen, in contrast to AEROBIC. Certain microbes are called anaerobes because they do not need oxygen.

analgesia   a deadening or absence of pain, without loss of consciousness. DRUGS such as ASPIRIN which produce this effect are termed analgesics.

anaphylaxis   a severe allergic reaction to the presence in the bloodstream of specific substances, characterized by spasm of the upper respiratory passages, hindering breathing and restricting blood flow, thus also lowering blood pressure. A person may for example be hypersensitive to penicillin or some other drug, to certain foods or to insect stings. Anaphylactic reaction may be catastrophic, with convulsions, unconsciousness, and death, unless there is prompt emergency treatment.

anastomosis   a connection between any two internal tubes or vessels, such as blood vessels.

anatomy   the study of the physical structure of living organisms. The word is also used to refer to the internal and external structure itself of an organism.

androgen   a general term for any SEX HORMONE of a male. The most important is TESTOSTERONE, which is responsible for the development of adult male characteristics during adolescence. Most androgens are produced by the testes; some are secreted by the adrenal glands.

anemia   a disorder in which the blood has fewer than the normal number of red BLOOD CELLS, or the cells are deficient in HEMOGLOBIN. The consequence is that the oxygen-transporting capability of the blood is reduced.

anesthetics   DRUGS that cause numbness or a loss of sensation; commonly used in conjunction with treatment that might otherwise be too painful to endure.

aneurin   another name for the VITAMIN thiamine.

aneurysm   a weakening in the wall of an ARTERY (or a vein), resulting in a bulge.

angiitis   inflammation of a blood vessel. Arteritis (inflammation of an artery), lymphangiitis (inflammation of a lymph vessel) and PHLEBITIS (inflammation of a vein) are all forms of angiitis.

angina pectoris   a painful, tight, dull or heavy feeling across the chest, which may spread to the neck, jaw, left shoulder and left arm. It is caused by a diminished supply of blood (and thus oxygen) to the heart muscle.

angiogram   a series of X-ray pictures of a blood vessel taken to establish whether or not it is of normal caliber or has abnormalities such as aneurysms or obstructions. The vessel is first injected with a radiopaque fluid that shows up on the X-ray film.

ankle   the joint between the lower leg and the foot.

ankylosing spondylitis   a chronic progressive condition in which the bones of the spine fuse together. The disorder almost exclusively attacks men aged between twenty and forty. Fusion begins usually at the base of the spine.

ankylosis   the stiffening of a joint caused by the fusing of the bones that form it. This may be the result of disease or it may be produced surgically to relieve pain.

anorexia nervosa   a psychological disorder, occurring mainly in adolescent girls, which is marked by a loathing of food expressed as an aversion to putting on weight. Subsequent wasting can be fatal.

anoxia a deficiency of oxygen in the body.

antacid an alkaline substance used medically to neutralize excess stomach acid.

antagonist any action or treatment that acts identically but in reverse or in opposition to a similar form of action or treatment — as in the action of one muscle that opposes the action of another muscle, or a drug that neutralizes another drug.

antenatal *see* PRENATAL.

anthelmintics DRUGS used to treat infestations by WORMS.

anthrax a rare bacterial infection that is passed on to humans through contact with contaminated animals or animal products. It is characterized by bluish-black skin masses and bleeding in the lungs and intestines, and may be fatal if left untreated.

antibiotics are antibacterial DRUGS originally developed from living organisms, such as molds and fungi. Most are now synthesized.

antibody any of a group of proteins produced by the body which protects it from disease or infection by "recognizing", interacting with, and so neutralizing or destroying, foreign substances such as invading bacteria. Anything that stimulates the production of antibodies is called an ANTIGEN. Antibodies are an essential part of the body's IMMUNE SYSTEM.

anticoagulants DRUGS that slow down or prevent the normal clotting of the blood.

anticonvulsants DRUGS used to prevent seizures or CONVULSIONS.

antidepressants psychoactive DRUGS used to relieve mental depression.

antidiuretic hormone (ADH) a hormone secreted by the PITUITARY GLAND. Its function is to control the reabsorption of water by the kidneys. It also causes contraction of the blood vessels, thus raising blood pressure.

antifungal drugs DRUGS used to treat fungal infections.

antigen any foreign substance or organism which stimulates the production of an ANTIBODY.

antihistamines DRUGS used to counteract the inflammatory actions of HISTAMINE.

antinauseants DRUGS used to prevent NAUSEA.

antipruritics DRUGS that prevent ITCHING.

antipyretics DRUGS that lower body temperature or reduce fever.

antiseptic something that destroys or prevents the growth of germs. Chemical antiseptics include certain DRUGS, household disinfectants and alcohol. Physical antiseptics include sunlight, radiation and heat.

antiserum a SERUM containing antibodies against a specific ANTIGEN. It is usually obtained from the blood of an animal or person exposed to or immunized against the ANTIGEN and which therefore contains the antibodies.

antispasmodics DRUGS that relieve muscle spasms, usually in smooth MUSCLE.

antitoxin an ANTIBODY to a specific poison, or toxin, usually originating from microorganisms such as bacteria or from the venom of certain animals. An antitoxin may be a constituent of an ANTISERUM.

antitussives DRUGS that inhibit coughing.

antivenin a specific ANTITOXIN used to treat poisoning by the venom of a particular animal, such as a snake.

anuria the inability to produce urine. It may be a symptom of diseased kidneys, a blockage in the urinary tract, or a lowering of blood pressure.

anus the orifice at the lower end of the RECTUM.

anxiety is a feeling of worry or fear in the apprehension of future events. When there is no legitimate basis for the anxiety it constitutes a psychological condition that may require professional psychiatric treatment.

aorta the largest ARTERY in the body. It carries blood from the HEART to the other major arteries.

aperient *see* LAXATIVE.

aphasia   a condition in which a person cannot speak. It is caused by temporary or permanent brain damage, most commonly following a STROKE.

aphrodisiac   any substance that stimulates sexual desire.

aphthous ulcer   *see* ULCER.

apocrine gland   a type of gland that loses part of the secreting cells with the secretion; examples include the mammary f ga3glands (breasts) and sweat glands, the groin and the armpit.

apoplexy   an outdated term for a STROKE.

appendectomy   the surgical removal of the APPENDIX, usually after APPENDICITIS has been diagnosed.

appendicitis   inflammation of the APPENDIX. Symptoms include severe pain around the navel and the right lower sector of the abdomen, fever, nausea and vomiting.

appendix   a hollow fingerlike projection of intestinal tissue, three to five inches long, arising off the CECUM.

aqueous humor   the watery fluid in the front of the eye, located between the cornea and the lens.

arachnoid membrane   the middle of three membranes that cover and protect the brain and spinal cord.

areola   the lightly pigmented ring surrounding the nipple of the breasts.

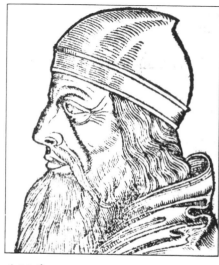

Aristotle

Aristotle (384–322 BC) ancient Greek philosopher who helped establish scientific method in biological sciences.

arm the upper limb between the shoulder and the wrist. Its framework is the humerus or upper arm bone and two lower bones, the radius and the ulna, which make up the forearm.

armpit (medical name axilla) the concave underside of the shoulder joint.

arrhythmia an irregularity in the heartbeat.

arteriogram X-ray image of an ARTERY.

arteriole a very small ARTERY.

arteriosclerosis hardening of the arteries. It occurs more commonly in middle and later life, as the arteries become naturally less elastic. The condition may be associated with ATHEROSCLEROSIS.

artery a blood vessel with muscular walls that carries blood away from the heart.

arthritis the general name for a group of disorders associated with inflammation of the joints, which may swell, become stiff and feel painful. Causes may include certain infections, metabolic disorders and complex immunological disorders (as in rheumatoid arthritis).

arthrodesis the artificial ANKYLOSIS (immobilization) of a joint.

articulation refers both to a joint and to the manner in which it moves or connects. The word is also used for the ability to connect words in speech.

artificial heart a mechanical device fitted with pumps and tubes, and located mostly outside the body, which takes over the functions of the heart while it is being operated on or until transplantation of a real heart from a donor can take place.

artificial insemination a technique for introducing SPERM into a woman's WOMB without sexual intercourse, generally after repeated failure to conceive.

artificial kidney a machine that performs kidney DIALYSIS.

artificial limb a synonym for a PROSTHESIS.

artificial respiration
============================

artificial respiration any method of restoring breathing to a person whose
breathing has stopped. There are several
first aid techniques for this purpose, including mouth-to-mouth resuscitation (the kiss
of life).

asbestosis a lung disorder caused by inhaling microscopic asbestos fibers over a
prolonged period. Symptoms of breathlessness may lead to ASTHMA and even to
lung cancer.

ascorbic acid the chemical name for
VITAMIN C.

asepsis a germ-free condition.

Asklepios the Greek god of medicine
and healing, known to the Romans as Aesculapius. Homer refers to him as a medical
expert present at the siege of Troy. His skill
in surgery and the use of drugs earned him
the title of the "Father of Medicine."

asphyxia lack of oxygen in the blood,
occurring when oxygen uptake by the
lungs is blocked externally or internally.

aspirator a suction instrument that re-
moves fluids from body cavities, such as
the lungs. It is also used by dentists to keep
the mouth dry and clean during treatment.

aspirin (acetylsalicylic acid) a colorless,
odorless DRUG with a bitter taste, commonly used as an analgesic (painkiller) and to
treat arthritis. It is becoming widely used
to treat certain heart conditions. Aspirin is
one of the oldest drugs known to humans.

asthma a disorder that produces spasms
and narrowing in the bronchial tubes; this
results in shortness of breath and characteristic wheezing on breathing out. Such
symptoms — of variable severity and
duration — may be brought on by INFEC-
TION or, more commonly, by an ALLERGY.
Asthmatic attacks may be associated with
emotional factors such as STRESS.

astigmatism an eye defect that
produces a blurring of vision. It is caused
by an abnormality in the shape of the cornea (the outer transparent layer) or the lens
of the eye.

astringent a substance that causes tissues and blood vessels to contract and helps
blood to coagulate. Common astringents
include alcohol, alum and silver nitrate.

ataxia loss of coordination in voluntary

muscular movement, usually from a neurological cause.

atheroma a fatty deposit on or fatty degeneration of part of the inner wall of an artery. This condition — a characteristic of ATHEROSCLEROSIS — impedes the blood flow and may, if the heart is involved, cause angina or INFARCTION.

atherosclerosis a condition in which fatty deposits (ATHEROMA) form inside a medium to large ARTERY and narrow the caliber of the vessel, thus impairing the blood flow. It is believed that excess CHOLESTEROL aggravates the condition, as do high blood pressure, cigarette smoking and continual stress.

athlete's foot a type of FUNGUS infection of the foot. The skin between the toes becomes soggy or scaly and peels away. The resulting lesion may itch painfully.

ATP (adenosine triphosphate) a NUCLEOTIDE (a compound formed of phosphoric acid, a sugar and a base) which, when converted to ADP, releases energy for muscle activity.

atrial fibrillation a disorder of the HEARTBEAT in which atrial contractions are rapid, irregular and out of synchronism with ventricular contractions.

atrial flutter is a disorder of the HEARTBEAT in which the contractions of the atria become very rapid (a rate of between 200 and 400 a minute).

atrium the name for each of the two left or right upper chambers of the HEART.

atrophy the wasting away of any part of the body.

atropine a drug that blocks PARASYMPATHETIC NERVOUS SYSTEM stimulation.

aura a psychophysical sensation — best known as a symptom of certain types of EPILEPSY.

auricle the part of the outer ear that extends from the head, also called the pinna.

auscultation listening to sounds within the body to determine the condition of the patient.

autism a psychological disorder that may appear in early childhood. The patient apparently withdraws from reality, and relates abnormally to people, objects and events.

autograft a tissue graft taken from one part of a patient's body for use on another part.

autoimmune disease any of a group of diseases caused by a breakdown in the IMMUNE SYSTEM. Normally this system distinguishes between the body's own tissues and "foreign" substances, and attacks the latter. In autoimmune disease, that distinction is not made and antibodies attack the body's own proteins.

autonomic nervous system that part of the nervous system that controls the involuntary functions of the body, such as glandular activity, and the heartbeat. It is divided into two systems: the SYMPATHETIC NERVOUS SYSTEM and the PARASYMPATHETIC NERVOUS SYSTEM.

autopsy *see* POST MORTEM.

axilla *see* ARMPIT.

axon the part of a NEURON through which impulses flow away from the NERVE CELL body.

B

Babbage, Charles (1792–1871) an English mathematician and mechanical genius who is regarded as the "father of the computer", modern versions of which are indispensable aids to medical research, diagnosis and treatment.

bacillus a rod-shaped BACTERIUM.

bacillus Calmette-Guérin the weakened form of tuberculosis bacillus that is used in BCG VACCINE.

backache a symptom of any one of several disorders, including SLIPPED DISK, LUMBAGO, uterine disorders, STRAIN and ARTHRITIS.

backbone the vertebral column or SPINE.

bacteremia describes the presence of bacteria in the blood.

bacterium, or microbe a one-celled microorganism. Bacteria thrive almost everywhere, and many types live within other living organisms. Some are helpful to body functions (such as digestion); others cause diseases.

bacteriophage a VIRUS that is parasitic on bacteria.

balance a learned skill related to the upright posture and sense of equilibrium of the body. It is controlled by hair cells in the three semicircular canals of the inner ear.

baldness, or alopecia partial or complete lack of hair.

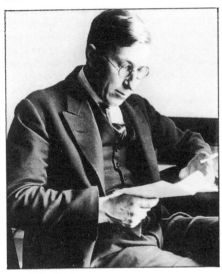

Banting, Frederick Grant (1891–1941) a Canadian physician mainly responsible for the isolation of INSULIN for use in the treatment of DIABETES in 1922. Banting was helped by John MACLEOD, who shared with him the 1923 Nobel Prize in physiology and medicine; both shared their honors with Charles BEST.

barbiturates DRUGS used as sedatives or general anesthetics.

barium a heavy metallic element; the basis for a flavored radiopaque mixture of barium sulfate and water swallowed by patients before X-ray examination of part of the alimentary canal. In a barium enema, a barium mixture is introduced into the rectum so that X-rays reveal the outline of the lower part of the intestines.

Barnard, Christiaan Neethling (1922–) South African surgeon who performed the world's first heart transplant in December 1967.

basal ganglia four centers of gray

matter deep inside the brain. They are associated with the unconscious control of voluntary movements.

basal metabolic rate (BMR)   the rate at which a person uses energy while at rest. It may be measured by the heat produced or by the amount of oxygen used over a short period.

basophil   a type of white BLOOD CELL with granules that are identified because they stain with basic dyes.

BCG vaccine (bacillus Calmette-Guérin) a preparation that contains a harmless strain of the live TUBERCULOSIS bacterium; it is used to immunize people against tuberculosis. It was named for Calmette and Guérin, the two French bacteriologists who first developed it.

Beaumont, William (1785–1853)   a US Army surgeon who pioneered the study of the physiology of digestion; he discovered that the acid secretion of the stomach was produced separately from the mucous secretions.

bedbug (*Cimex lectularius*)   a small, wingless, bloodsucking insect that may infest bedding. Its bites can cause painful swelling or itching.

bedpan   a shallow vessel used to collect urine and feces from bedridden patients.

bedsore, or pressure sore   an ulcerated skin condition that affects bedridden patients who are unable to move unaided in bed. The sore forms in pressure areas on which the patient has been lying for too long a time.

bed-wetting (enuresis)   a condition common among young children. Total bladder control is usually achieved by the age of four or five.

behaviorism   a school of psychology based on the concept of the CONDITIONED REFLEX. It propounds that psychic events are the results of the functions of nerves and glands, and that the only acceptable subjects for psychological study are the objective (visible, measurable) aspects of behavior.

behavior therapy   a means of modifying a patient's antisocial behavior by means of treatment involving a series of rewards and punishments.

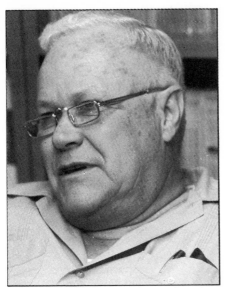

Beidler, Lloyd (1922–) an American physiologist and one of the world's greatest experts on TASTE. In the 1950s, Beidler and his colleagues established that each single chemoreceptor cell can react to different substances, for example to both salt and sucrose (sugar) and so are not specific, as previously thought.

Békésy, Georg von (1899–1972) a Hungarian-born American who won the Nobel Prize in physiology and medicine in 1961. He discovered that different sound frequencies are analyzed by the COCHLEA at different locations along its basilar membrane.

Bell, Charles (1774–1842) a Scottish physician who, in his *Idea of a New Anatomy of the Brain* (1811), clearly distinguished between the functions of motor and sensory nerves, and claimed to be the first to do so, although this was disputed by François MAGENDIE.

Bell's palsy the frequently reversible paralysis of some of the muscles of the face. It stems from malfunction of the facial nerve that supplies the muscles on one side of the face. The effect — a drooping of the mouth and one eyelid — often goes unnoticed by the patient. The cause is generally unknown.

bends the common name for DECOMPRESSION SICKNESS, usually a consequence of deep-sea diving.

benign describes a tumor that does not spread to other sites, or a mild disease; it contrasts with MALIGNANT.

beriberi a tropical disease caused by lack of VITAMIN B, (thiamine). Symptoms include stiffness in the legs, paralysis and pain.

Bernard, Claude (1813–1878) a French scientist who first deduced the intestines' role in digestion. He also discovered the importance of the PANCREAS in breaking down fat. He demonstrated that carbon monoxide poisoning occurs because this gas combines with hemoglobin to deprive the body of oxygen, thus leading to the condition of ASPHYXIA.

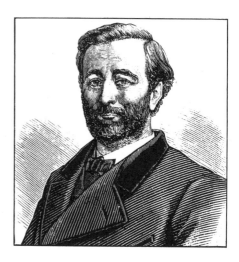

Bert, Paul (1833–1886) a French physiologist who has been called the founder of aerospace medicine. He was the first to study the behaviour of blood under a range of gas pressures, and his systematic study of the DECOMPRESSION SICKNESS suffered by divers, known as the bends, helped to make possible the exploration of ocean depths, as well as space.

Best, Charles Herbert (1899–) a Canadian physiologist who, in 1922, helped Frederick BANTING to isolate INSULIN for use in the treatment of DIABETES.

beta-blocker the abbreviation for beta adrenergic blocking agents — DRUGS that inhibit SYMPATHETIC NERVOUS SYSTEM stimulation, and so help reduce heart rate and BLOOD PRESSURE.

biceps the two-headed muscle at the front of the upper arm, used as a FLEXOR of the arm.

Bichat, Marie François Xavier (1771–1802) a French anatomist, pathologist, and physiologist whose recognition that the human body is made up of tissues laid the foundations for modern HISTOLOGY, and revolutionized the study of disease.

bifocals   a type of EYEGLASSES used by people who suffer from either MYOPIA or HYPEROPIA.

bile   the bitter, green-yellow fluid produced by the LIVER from the breakdown of red blood cells, stored in the GALL BLADDER and released into the small intestine to aid the digestion of fats.

biliary colic   is abdominal pain caused by GALLSTONES or infection in the BILE system.

Billroth, Theodore   (1829–1894) a celebrated German surgeon who made valuable contributions to military surgery, histology and pathology. He established the modern concept of writing up reports on operations and instigated a five-year follow-up of such cases.

BMR   *see* BASAL METABOLIC RATE.

biofeedback   a technique that uses electronic measurement of patients' pulse rate, perspiration and BLOOD PRESSURE while they attempt to consciously control bodily functions that are generally regarded as involuntary. By monitoring such functions, each patient can see the results of his or her efforts and, when successful, endeavor to repeat them.

biomechanics   the science of the mechanical functions of parts of living organisms.

bionic limb   a sophisticated PROSTHESIS.

biopsy   a procedure by which a small sample of body tissue is removed from a patient (possibly under local anesthetic) in order to make a diagnosis or to monitor a course of treatment.

biotin   part of the VITAMIN B complex.

birth control   *see* CONTRACEPTION.

birthmark   a skin blemish, usually pigmented, present at or appearing shortly after birth.

bisexuality   a state of being attracted sexually to both men and women, as distinct from HETEROSEXUALITY or HOMOSEXUALITY.

black eye discoloration of the skin and swelling around the eye, representing a BRUISE of the soft tissues around the ORBIT. It usually follows a blow that ruptures minute blood vessels in this region.

blackhead, or comedo a plug of hardened SEBUM in a sebaceous gland in the SKIN.

blackout temporary unconsciousness (or, rarely, loss of vision) caused by disturbed or inadequate blood flow to the brain.

bladder the organ that collects and holds urine passed to it by the ureters from the kidneys. It releases urine through a tube called the urethra.

blastocyst an early stage in the development of an EMBRYO, when a fertilized OVUM has divided to form a fluid-filled ball, its surface made up of about fifty cells. It is at this stage that IMPLANTATION occurs.

bleeding blood loss; the common name for HEMORRHAGE.

blepharitis inflammation of the eyelids.

blindness a partial or total loss of vision from one or both eyes.

blind spot a small oval-shaped area at the back of the eye where the RETINA coincides with the OPTIC NERVE, and there are no light-sensitive cells.

blister a localized superficial accumulation of SERUM under the skin; it results from damage to the outer layers of the skin, for example from friction, inflammation or burning.

blood the fluid that fills the vessels of the cardiovascular system and forms the primary internal transportation system of the body. It consists of PLASMA and various types of BLOOD CELLS.

blood cells various types of cells within the blood. Red cells, or ERYTHROCYTES, are chiefly concerned with the transportation of oxygen and carbon dioxide through the body. Small clear PLATELETS are important in blood clotting. White cells or corpuscles, also called LEUKOCYTES, include BASOPHILS, LYMPHOCYTES, MONOCYTES and NEUTROPHILS, all of which help combat infection.

blood clot a mass of congealed blood.

Surface clotting helps to stop bleeding after an injury and is an important defense mechanism. A clot in a blood vessel, however, is called a THROMBUS and can obstruct the normal flow of blood.

blood count a blood test that determines the number of red blood cells, white blood cells, and platelets in a person's blood from an analysis of a small sample. It is a valuable test: most diseases affect the blood count in characteristic ways.

blood group a classification of a person's blood according to the presence or absence of certain proteins in the red blood cells. Categorization is essential to successful blood TRANSFUSION. In the ABO system there are four groups: A, B, AB, and O. In the Rhesus system there are six types based on Rhesus positive (Rh+) and Rhesus negative (Rh−).

blood poisoning (septicemia or toxemia) a general term for any medical condition resulting from the circulation of bacteria or poisonous substances in the blood.

blood pressure a measurement of the force with which blood presses against the wall of a blood vessel. It is usually measured in an artery in the arm, the pressure during (systolic) and after (diastolic) the pumping action of a heartbeat.

blood sugar the sugar in the form of GLUCOSE present in blood. Blood sugar levels are highest after eating. Abnormally high or low blood sugar levels that persist may be symptoms of a metabolic disorder such as DIABETES MELLITUS.

blood tests analyze the chemical or physical composition of a person's blood. Common tests include those for BLOOD COUNT, BLOOD GROUP, BLOOD SUGAR or ERYTHROCYTE SEDIMENTATION RATE.

blood transfusion *see* TRANSFUSION.

blood vessels ARTERIES, CAPILLARIES, or VEINS.

blue baby a newborn whose blood is deficient in oxygen. As a result, the skin takes on a bluish tinge (cyanosis). The cause is usually a congenital heart defect requiring surgical correction.

blushing usually the result of embarrassment; a sudden reddening of the skin, brought on by increased blood flow in the skin capillaries.

BONES

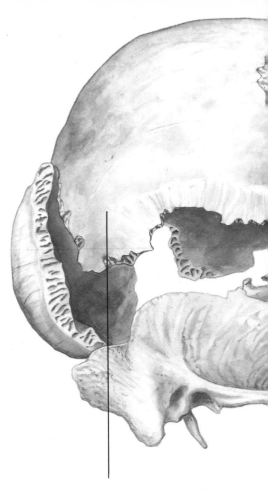

Bones enclosing brain

Lower jaw (mandible) ——————

Bones can mend themselves when broken or fractured. Healing begins with the formation of a large blood clot around the break. Secondly, a cuff of cartilage called a callus forms around the break, to stabilize it. New bone then grows out into the callus until the break is healed.

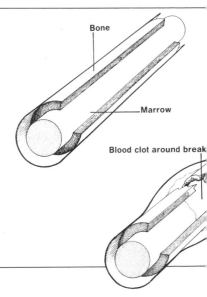

Bone

Marrow

Blood clot around break

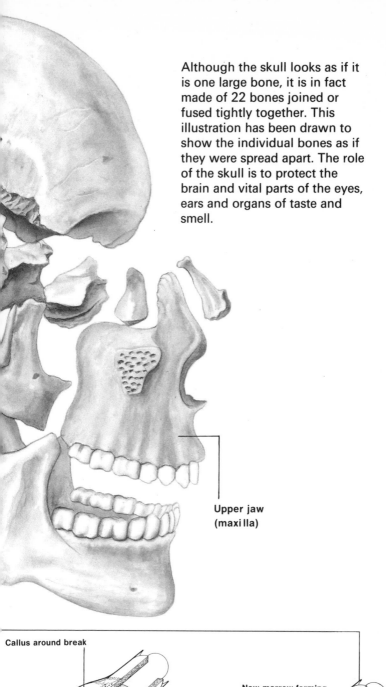

Although the skull looks as if it is one large bone, it is in fact made of 22 bones joined or fused tightly together. This illustration has been drawn to show the individual bones as if they were spread apart. The role of the skull is to protect the brain and vital parts of the eyes, ears and organs of taste and smell.

Upper jaw
(maxilla)

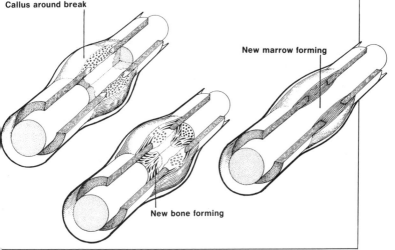

Callus around break

New marrow forming

New bone forming

BMR

BMR *see* BASAL METABOLIC RATE.

body odor medically known as brom-hidrosis, a smell that results from the action of bacteria in stale sweat on the skin.

body temperature *see* TEMPERATURE, or FEVER.

boil, or furuncle a painful, swollen infection in a sweat gland or hair root. Boils are caused by bacteria and in severe cases can lead to BLOOD POISONING.

bone the hard calcium-based tissue formed from CARTILAGE that composes the bones of the skeleton.

bone graft the transplantation of a healthy piece of bone from one area in a patient's body to replace or help regenerate a damaged bone.

bone marrow the gelatinous tissue that fills the hollow cavities of bones. Red marrow is a major site of the production of red blood cells and hemoglobin. Fatty yellow marrow occurs principally in the shafts of long bones.

booster a supplementary dose of an inoculation or VACCINE to extend or increase the original protection.

Borlaug, Norman E. (1914–   ) an American plant pathologist who was awarded the Nobel Peace Prize in 1970 for his work in the genetic improvement of varieties of wheat.

bottle-feeding a necessary procedure to provide a baby with food when the mother chooses not to supply breast milk, when the milk supply is inadequate, or when the baby refuses her nipple. The prescription for the contents of the bottle, called the formula, usually consists mainly of fresh or powdered cow's milk mixed with water and sugar.

botulism a rare but serious type of FOOD POISONING.

bowel *see* INTESTINE.

bowlegs legs that curve outward leaving a space between the knees when the feet are together. In adults this may be due to OSTEOMALACIA; in children it used to occur as a result of RICKETS.

Bowman, William (1816–1892) an English ophthalmic surgeon and pioneer histologist who was the first to discover that the cup-shaped end of a kidney tubule (since named BOWMAN'S CAPSULE) forms part of the tube that drains urine.

Bowman's capsule the end of the renal tubule that surrounds each GLOMERULUS of the KIDNEY; together these constitute the structure in which renal filtration occurs.

bradycardia a very slow heartbeat with a pulse rate of less than about fifty or sixty a minute. It may be the result of heart block or the effect of a drug.

Braille raised dots on paper that can be "read" by touch.

brain the mass of neural tissue enclosed and protected by the CRANIUM, and the principal element of the central nervous system.

brainstem the central part of the brain, comprising all parts except the CEREBRUM and CEREBELLUM.

brain waves electrical impulses in the brain. These may be recorded by a machine called an ELECTROENCEPHALOGRAPH (EEG).

bran the coarse husks of cereal grains. Its high fiber content makes it useful as the roughage necessary in the diet to protect against intestinal disorders.

breast the front and upper part of the chest. The term is also used for the mammary gland of a woman, in whom it is the milk-producing organ, which develops at puberty, but produces milk only after CHILDBIRTH. Female breasts consist of milk glands, milk ducts and fatty tissue. Milk ducts lead to the nipple, from which milk emerges during LACTATION.

breast bone *see* STERNUM.

breast cancer the most common CANCER affecting women, of whom it affects some 7 per cent. It may be fairly easily detected in its early stages by careful and regular self-examination (palpation); such early detection is associated with a greater likelihood of cure.

breast-feeding (nursing or suckling) feeding a baby from the mother's breast. Natural milk production (LACTATION) coincides with the birth of a baby.

breast lump a lump in the tissue of the

breast which may be discovered during the process of regular self-examination. It may be a cyst or a benign growth; sometimes it is a sign of BREAST CANCER. A breast lump should always be examined by a physician.

breathing the physical inhalation and exhalation of air that occurs in RESPIRATION.

breathlessness normal after exertion. But when labored breathing (dyspnea) occurs at rest, it can be a symptom of lung disorders such as ASTHMA or PNEUMONIA; it may also be caused by HEART DISEASE or ANEMIA.

breech birth occurs when a baby is born feet or buttocks first, instead of head first.

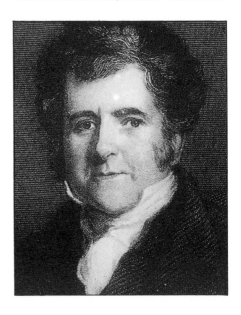

Bright, Richard (1789−1858) an English physician who was the first to diagnose and describe chronic GLOMERULONEPHRITIS, which became known as Bright's disease.

Broca, Paul (1824−1880) a French surgeon and anthropologist who was the first to show that one specific region of the brain may be responsible for controlling a specific activity. He discovered the seat of articulate speech in the brain.

bromhidrosis *see* BODY ODOR.

bronchi the two branches (each called a bronchus) of the air passage from the TRACHEA into the lungs.

bronchial dilators DRUGS that relax the bronchi to improve the breathing of patients with chronic chest disorders.

bronchiectasis   a chronic disease of the air passages to the LUNGS which dilate and tend to fill with PUS.

bronchiole   a small air passage in the lung. Bronchioles are the smaller branches of the bronchial "tree".

bronchitis   inflammation of the air passages to the LUNGS. Acute or chronic, it is commonly caused by an infection. Symptoms include a persistent cough and difficulty in breathing.

bronchogenic carcinoma   *see* LUNG CANCER.

bronchoscope   an instrument used to examine the TRACHEA or BRONCHI.

bruise (medical name, contusion)   an injury, usually caused by a blow or by pressure on the surface of the body, that does not break the skin. A purplish discoloration just below the skin results from the restricted escape of blood from small blood vessels into the soft tissues.

Brunner, Jerome Seymour (1915–)   an American psychologist and educationalist who identifies three stages in cognitive development: the "enactive" (a baby does what he or she thinks); the "iconic" (images replace physical action); and the "symbolic" (sensory images are replaced by verbal expression).

bubonic plague   an acute bacterial disease, often leading to PNEUMONIA. Characterized by highly swollen lymph nodes, it is usually transmitted to human beings by the bite of a flea which carries the disease from an infected rat.

bulimia   insatiable appetite. It is sometimes caused by brain damage; most other cases have a psychological origin.

bunion   a painful swollen deformity of the big toe. Pressure on the joint inflames the BURSA there, which swells and causes the toe to thicken and turn toward the other toes.

burn   an injury to the tissues caused by heat, electricity, chemicals, friction or radiation. Burns are classified according to the extent of the damage done to the skin. A first-degree burn turns the skin red without blisters. Second-degree goes deeper, with very red skin and blistering. Third-degree destroys the skin — both

EPIDERMIS and DERMIS — and leaves an open wound.

bursa a small, fluid-filled pouch that provides lubrication and flexibility where bones, tendons or ligaments move against each other.

bursitis the painful inflammation of a BURSA. Symptoms of bursitis also include swelling and tenderness of the affected joint. The knee and the elbow are most commonly affected.

by-pass *see* CARDIOPULMONARY BY-PASS.

C

calcaneus the heel bone of the foot.

calciferol a synthetic form of VITAMIN D, known as vitamin D$_2$.

calcification the normal or abnormal hardening of body tissues as a result of the deposit of calcium salts.

calcitonin a HORMONE secreted by the THYROID gland. With PARATHORMONE, from the PARATHYROID glands, it regulates calcium metabolism.

calcium a metallic element that occurs in the body in compound form, almost always as calcium phosphate. Calcium is essential to health, making up most of the mineral part of bones and teeth. An adequate calcium level in the blood is necessary for the proper functioning of nerves and muscles. Milk, eggs and beans are good dietary sources of calcium.

calculus, or stone an abnormal, hard, stonelike mass that may form in any of various cavities in organs of the body.

callus an area of tissue that has roughened and thickened, usually from rubbing. A CORN is a type of callus.

calorie a unit of energy measurement used in dietetics to express the amount of energy released by the consumption of various foods.

cancer a growth of abnormal cells, often in the form of a TUMOR, in which the cells are MALIGNANT and tend to spread to new sites (METASTASIS), where they damage or destroy organs or tissues.

candidiasis a fungal infection of the MUCOUS MEMBRANES or the skin. Commonly affecting the mouth and throat, it also attacks other areas such as the genitals.

canine one of the four slightly pointed TEETH between the INCISORS and the MOLARS.

canker sore a small painful sore, probably caused by a virus, most commonly on the mouth or lips.

cap, contraceptive another name for the contraceptive DIAPHRAGM.

CAPD stands for CONTINUOUS AMBULATORY PERITONEAL DIALYSIS, a sophisticated form of home DIALYSIS.

capillaries microscopic blood vessels, often little wider than a blood cell.

carbohydrate one of the three main types of substance (together with proteins and fats) that make up food. It comprises only carbon, hydrogen and oxygen, and enters the bloodstream after digestion as a simple sugar such as glucose.

carbon dioxide a gas, present in the atmosphere, that is formed in the body tissues as a waste product of metabolism. The blood carries it to the LUNGS from which it is expelled in breathing.

carbon monoxide a poisonous, flammable, colorless gas. Present in car exhausts, it binds firmly to hemoglobin in the blood and can prove fatal if too much is inhaled because it blocks oxygen uptake by red blood cells.

carbuncle a type of severe BOIL.

carcinogen any substance that causes CANCER.

carcinoma a type of CANCER originating in epithelial cells.

cardiac of or concerning the HEART.

cardiac arrest occurs when the heart stops

cardiac cycle the period from the start of one heart beat to the start of the next. It includes the SYSTOLE (the forceful contraction of the ventricles which pumps the blood out of the heart into the AORTA), and the DIASTOLE (when the ventricles relax and refill with blood). the normal cycle lasts about four-fifths of a second.

cardiac massage *see* CARDIOPULMONARY RESUSCITATION.

cardiac muscle the specialized involuntary muscle of which the HEART is composed.

cardiac pacemaker the PACEMAKER that regulates the CARDIAC CYCLE.

cardiogram *see* ELECTROCARDIOGRAM.

cardiology the study of the heart and its disorders.

cardiopulmonary by-pass a technique by which the blood circulation is maintained during heart surgery. Blood returning to the heart is rerouted instead to a HEART-LUNG MACHINE which both oxygenates the blood and pumps it into the circulation.

cardiopulmonary circulation the circulation of blood between the heart and the lungs.

cardiopulmonary resuscitation (CPR) a method of keeping a person alive who has experienced cardiac arrest, respiratory arrest, or both, by a combination of heart massage and the mouth-to-mouth resuscitation technique known generally as the kiss of life.

cardiovascular system the general name for the circulatory system, the arteries and veins, through which blood is pumped by the heart.

caries *see* TOOTH DECAY.

carotene the chemical name for the red pigment, found in certain vegetables (particularly carrots), that is the dietary precursor of VITAMIN A.

carotid artery one of the major arteries carrying blood from the aorta to the head.

carpal tunnel syndrome a painful disorder of the wrist, often caused by overactivity, that results in numbness, tingling or tenderness in the hand and fingers. It results from compression of the median nerve by the band of cartilage around the wrist, possibly from inflammation of the carpal tunnel beneath this band.

carpus the bones at the wrist.

Carrel, Alexis (1873 – 1944) a French surgeon and biologist who pioneered the transplantation of organs and the suturing (stitching together) of blood vessels. Together with aviator Charles Lindbergh he designed a perfusion pump (the forerunner of apparatus used today in major heart surgery). In World War I, with Henry Dakind, he devised an antiseptic for treating infected wounds. In 1912 he was awarded the Nobel Prize for physiology and medicine.

carrier   a person who, without showing any visible symptoms of a disorder, nevertheless "carries" it in the body or genes and can pass it on to other persons. This may occur with such diseases as TYPHOID and AIDS, or with congenital disorders such as HEMOPHILIA. An animal or insect (such as a mosquito) which transmits disease to humans is generally known as a vector.

car sickness   a form of TRAVEL SICKNESS.

cartilage   the tough, but flexible, tissue that covers the ends of bones where they form moving joints. It also forms structures such as the nose and external ears.

cast   a hard mold of a part of the body, usually made from plaster. It is used to immobilize that part during healing, most commonly of a FRACTURE. It is a specialized type of SPLINT.

castration   is the removal of the reproductive organs; the term usually refers to the removal of a male's testicles. This leads to sterility.

CAT   the acronym for COMPUTERIZED AXIAL TOMOGRAPHY (a CAT scan).

cataract   a clouding of the lens of the eye. It is a common disorder of the elderly, in whom the dimness, if left untreated, may progress to total blindness.

catarrh   excessive secretion of mucus from the nose and throat, usually resulting from an upper respiratory tract infection (such as the common cold).

catatonia   thought to be a form of SCHIZOPHRENIA: the patient becomes rigid and seems to be in a stupor, although such symptoms are interrupted with occasional outbursts of excitement.

catecholamines   biologically active chemicals that produce the effects of stress on the cardiovascular and nervous systems, on the metabolic rate, the smooth muscle, and on body temperature.

catharsis in PSYCHOANALYSIS, the release of neurotic tension associated with recall of the cause of a psychoneurosis.

cathartic a strong LAXATIVE.

catheter a flexible plastic or rubber tube that may be inserted into a body vessel or cavity, such as the bladder, in order to inject or withdraw fluids.

Cattell, James McKeen (1860–1944) a leading American psychologist who investigated the interval between stimulus and reaction and the effect on it of varying the intensity of the stimulus. Much later, in Philadelphia, he devised and carried out tests for measuring the mental abilities of students.

cauterization, or cautery the destruction of abnormal or damaged tissue by means of electricity, chemicals, a laser or a very hot or very cold instrument. Most of these processes also have the effect of sealing up small ruptured blood vessels.

cecum the pouch that forms the first section of the large intestine, located where the small intestine joins the colon. The APPENDIX is attached to the cecum.

celiac disease a chronic disorder of the small intestine caused by sensitivity to gluten, a protein present in wheat and other cereals. As a result, normal absorption of food, especially fats, is prevented.

cell the smallest unit of living matter. All living tissues are built from cells. The cell is made up of a nucleus surrounded by jelly-like cytoplasm, various cellular bodies (organelles), and an outer membrane.

cellulose a CARBOHYDRATE on which human digestive processes have no effect. A major constituent of leaves, and similar to starch in structure, it is also present in green vegetables and fruits. Because it is indigestible, it constitutes part of the dietary fiber that helps in the elimination of waste products.

central nervous system consists of the BRAIN and SPINAL CORD.**cerebellum** part of the BRAIN.

cerebral hemispheres the two halves of the CEREBRUM.

cerebral palsy a general term for various conditions, characterized by some lack of muscle control, that result from damage to the brain at or around the time of birth. In some cases it may be associated with mental retardation.

cerebrospinal fluid a clear, colorless liquid that bathes the spinal cord and the brain. It serves as a protective cushion and barrier for the central nervous system.

cerebrovascular accident *see* STROKE.

cerebrum the two large lobes (hemispheres) of the forebrain that give the human BRAIN its characteristic shape, size and appearance.

cerumen the medical name for EARWAX.

cervical cancer a malignant tumor in the CERVIX or neck of the womb — one of the commonest types of cancers in women. If diagnosed early, by means of a CERVICAL SMEAR TEST, it can frequently be successfully treated.

cervical erosion a condition in women in which the lining of the CERVIX of the womb is eroded away by bacterial invasion. Although susceptible to ulceration, it is not in itself serious.

cervical smear test, or Pap test a simple and painless method of checking for potentially cancerous cells in the tissues of the CERVIX of the womb at an early stage. It entails collecting a small specimen of cervical cells from the cervix and examining the specimen using a microscope.

cervical vertebrae the seven small bones that form the neck, making up the upper part of the spinal column.

cervix an abbreviation of cervix uteri, the neck of the womb, which projects into the vagina. The term cervix is also used for the "neck" of any organ.

chancre a painless ulcer that is a symptom of SYPHILIS. It occurs usually on the penis in men and on the vulva in women.

chancroid a condition in which the most significant symptom is a small, red soft sore on the genitals that resembles a syphilitic CHANCRE. It is a highly infectious SEXUALLY-TRANSMITTED DISEASE.

Charcot, Jean-Martin (1825–1893) a French neurologist who is regarded as the

CELLS

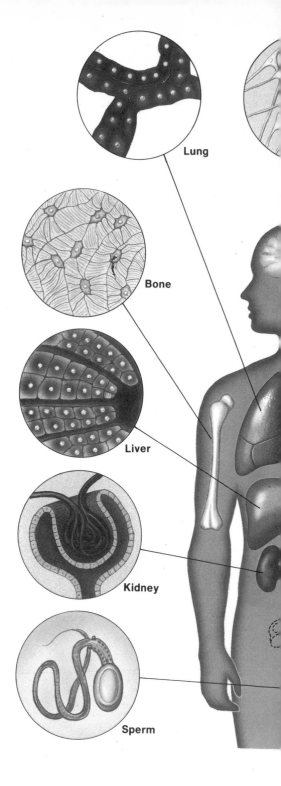

Lung

Bone

Liver

Kidney

Sperm

The diagram illustrates 11 of the hundreds of different types of body cells.

The egg is one of the largest cells and the one from which, once fertilized by a sperm cell, all the other cells are derived.

Epithelial or skinlike cells cover many spaces inside and outside the body, including th airspaces in the lungs and the kidneys' minute filters.

There are many different types of gland cell. Pancreas cells produce either digestive enzymes or the hormone insu which is vital to sugar metabolism. Liver cells are als

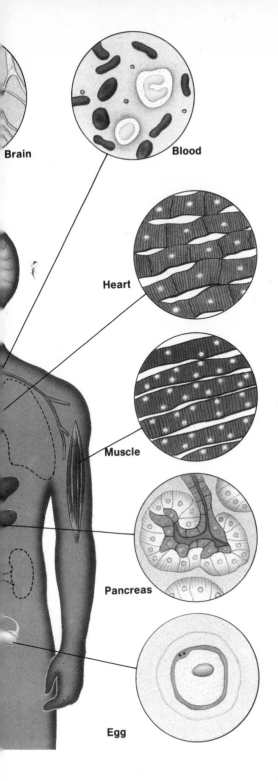

Brain

Blood

Heart

Muscle

Pancreas

Egg

volved in metabolic
ocesses.
Blood is a fluid tissue
ntaining red and white cells;
ese have different structures
d functions.
Nerve cells and muscle cells
e both elongate in shape.
uscle cells vary in structure

according to the roles they
perform: those of the heart have
a branched form compared with
other types.

Bone cells comprise the
skeleton.

founder of modern neurology. He was the first to describe neurological conditions such as tabes dorsalis, a symptom of advanced SYPHILIS, and MULTIPLE SCLEROSIS. He also provided a scientific understanding of hysteria, and made much use of HYPNOTISM in his treatment.

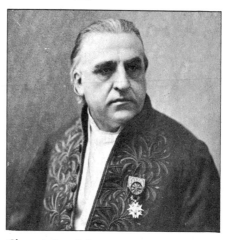

Charcot, Jean-Martin

cheiropompholyx a disease of the skin characterized by small blisters on the hands and feet.

chemotherapy the use of DRUGS to treat disease. Certain chemotherapeutic agents, particularly those used in the treatment of CANCER, are so powerful that marked adverse SIDE EFFECTS are inevitable.

Cheyne-Stokes breathing an extremely uneven breathing pattern, often found in the terminal stages of a disease.

chiasma an anatomical word for a crossing. The term usually refers to the optic chiasma, where the optic nerves cross on their way from each eye to the brain.

chickenpox (medical name, varicella) infection by a virus of the HERPES family, common in children. Highly contagious, although not considered serious, it is marked by a rash on the skin of small pimples, initially red but then colorless, which thereafter become scabs. The same virus causes SHINGLES in adults.

chilblain local swelling, reddening and pain or itching of the fingers, toes, ears or nose. The condition results from poor circulation.

childbirth the processes of LABOR and parturition that conclude a PREGNANCY.

chiropractic an unorthodox method of therapy which consists mainly of spinal manipulation. It is based on the premise that all disorders stem from the malfunctioning of the nervous system.

chlamydia a microorganism that has features of both a VIRUS and a BACTERIUM. Species of chlamydia cause various infections, among them the eye disease trachoma, a serious infection similar to CONJUNCTIVITIS.

chloasma localized light-brown skin discolorations that occur in certain conditions but are particularly associated with pregnancy or the use of contraceptive pills.

choking difficulty in breathing or inability to breathe caused by a blocking of the breathing passages (often by food or vomit). It can cause death from suffocation. An emergency treatment is the HEIMLICH MANEUVER.

cholecystectomy the surgical removal of the GALL BLADDER.

cholecystitis acute or chronic inflammation of the GALL BLADDER. Gallstones (CALCULI) are nearly always the cause of the acute form. They are not necessarily present in the chronic form. Some symptoms are pain, belching, shaking chills and vomiting. Treatment is usually by CHOLECYSTECTOMY.

cholelithiasis the presence of gallstones in the GALL BLADDER.

cholera acute gastrointestinal infection caused by a vibrio bacillus. Symptoms include diarrhea, severe fluid loss, cramps, dehydration and collapse, leading to death unless adequate fluid replacement can be maintained.

cholesterol a constituent of fatty foods. It is both manufactured in the body and taken in animal-derived food such as milk, butter and eggs. High levels in the blood may promote arterial disease.

Chomsky, Noam (1928–) an American psycholinguist who dramatically reshaped the modern study of verbal articulation.

chorea a symptom of various diseases that may affect the nervous system. It is marked by involuntary muscular twitching of the face and limbs. The two main types are HUNTINGTON'S CHOREA and SYDENHAM'S CHOREA.

chorion the outermost membrane that envelops the FETUS in the WOMB.

chorionic villus sampling a method of checking during pregnancy that a fetus is not developing abnormally. The CHORION has thousands of microscopic projections called villi. A small sample removed from these can reveal irregularities that may indicate genetic abnormalities in the fetus.

choroiditis inflammation of the choroid (the middle coat of the eyeball). The symptoms tend to be a gradual blurring of vision, with intermittent flashes of light.

chromosome one of a number of threadlike structures in the nucleus of a cell. It stores genetic information and by replication carries it from one generation of cells to the next. By this means genetic traits are also inherited by children from their parents.

chronic persistent, without any rapid change; it is applied to any disorder that lingers for a long time.

chyle a fatty product of digestion, formed in the tiny lymphatic vessels (lacteals) of intestinal VILLI. It passes from there through the LYMPHATIC SYSTEM into the blood.

chylomicron a microscopic fatty particle that enters the blood as a product of digestion and fat absorption.

chyme the semi-liquid mixture of food in the stomach and small intestine that is in the process of being digested.

cicatrix the medical synonym for a SCAR.

cilia microscopic hairlike growths that project from many body cells. In wavelike motion their rhythmic beating helps to sweep along particles in fluid or mucus.

circadian rhythm the regular daily cycle of certain bodily activities, such as sleeping. An internal "biological clock" is presumed to be responsible for this rhythm.

circumcision the removal of part of the FORESKIN. It is a religious rite among Jews and Muslims, but may alternatively be carried out for hygienic reasons.

cirrhosis a chronic disease of the LIVER in which healthy cells are destroyed and replaced by fatty or fibrous tissue. It is associated with liver damage from toxins such as alcohol or disease such as HEPATITIS.

claudication the medical term for limping or lameness, usually caused by vascular disease of the leg.

claustrophobia an abnormal fear of being enclosed.

clavicle the anatomical name for the collarbone.

clawfoot a deformity of the foot caused by nerve injury. It is marked by an abnormally high arch and contracted toes.

clawhand a deformity of the hand in which the fingers are permanently tensed like a claw. It is usually the result of an injury to the nerves.

cleft palate a congenital defect involving a split in the roof of the mouth; often accompanied by a similar split in the upper lip (HARELIP). The condition can usually be surgically repaired.

climacteric in a woman, the time of life at which the bodily changes of the MENOPAUSE take place.

clitoris a small, highly sensitive, erectile structure located at the front of the VULVA. It plays a major part in female ORGASM.

clot *see* BLOOD CLOT.

clotting the coagulation of blood; the natural process by which the body stops bleeding and promotes wound-healing. When a blood vessel is damaged, fibrinogen in the blood PLASMA forms a web of fine fibrin threads, in which blood cells and PLATELETS are entangled to form a plug (a clot) over the wound. Abnormal clotting within a blood vessel may cause THROMBOSIS; any deficiency in the clotting process may lead to HEMOPHILIA.

clubfoot a deformity of the foot, existing from birth. The bones are usually twisted, and the muscles and tendons stretched or shortened. Treatment consists of manipulation and a corrective brace; surgery is sometimes helpful.

coagulation *see* CLOTTING.

coccus a spherical or egg-shaped BAC-TERIUM.

coccyx the group of four small, joined vertebrae at the base of the spine.

cochlea the coiled, tubular structure in the inner EAR.

coil a common name for an IN-TRAUTERINE DEVICE (IUD) used in CON-TRACEPTION.

cold (medical name, coryza) an infectious disease of the respiratory tract, characterized by a running or stuffy nose, headache, and cough. Colds are caused by constantly evolving viruses, and a permanent cure has yet to be found.

coldsore a small sore on or near the lips, and sometimes in the genital region. It is caused by a virus (herpes simplex) and often manifests itself during other minor infections, hence its other name, fever sore.

colic spasms of acute abdominal pain. In babies this is not unusual, and is caused by cramps or gas in the stomach or intestine. In adults it may result from gallstones, inflammation of the gall bladder (biliary colic), or stones in the kidney (renal colic).

colitis inflammation of the COLON. There are two main types: the relatively mild mucous colitis, and the potentially more serious ulcerative colitis.

collagen a tough, fibrous protein that is a major constituent of CONNECTIVE TISSUE.

collagen disease a group of allied disorders affecting the CONNECTIVE TISSUE.

collarbone *see* CLAVICLE.

colon the lower part of the intestine.

colonic irrigation the technical description of an ENEMA.

color blindness an inherited defect of vision in which the patient is partly or totally unable to distinguish between certain colors, most commonly red and green.

colostomy an opening made surgically in the wall of the abdomen in order that waste products may be discharged through it directly from the COLON. A special renewable colostomy bag is ordinarily provided to cover the opening and collect the waste products.

colostrum the first secretion from a mother's breasts just before and after childbirth. It is a milklike substance consisting of serum, white blood cells, and antibodies.

colposcopy internal examination of the vagina and cervix by means of a specifically designed instrument (colposcope).

coma a state of unconsciousness in which there is no reaction to external stimuli. Regarded as a temporary condition, it may nevertheless last for years.

comedo *see* BLACKHEAD.

Comfort, Alex (1920–) a British gerontologist studying the processes of aging, who combats modern society's condemnation of senior citizens as mentally and physically infirm. His book, *The Biology of Senescence*, has become a standard textbook on the aging process.

comminuted fracture a type of complex FRACTURE in which a bone is crushed by a severe blow.

complex a term used in PSYCHO-ANALYSIS to describe a group of strongly emotive feelings that influence a person's behavior although they may conflict with the conscious mind. Psychoanalysts believe that such feelings may be repressed, leading to worry and subsequent guilt, which may thereafter result in mental illness.

compound fracture a type of FRACTURE in which the skin is broken and the bone exposed.

computerized axial tomography (CAT) an X-RAY technique used to examine the body's internal tissues. A device called a CAT scanner X-rays sections of the body from various angles. These are combined and analyzed by a computer to produce a cross-sectional image of the subject.

conception the FERTILIZATION of an ovum by a sperm.

concussion temporary loss of consciousness resulting from a blow to the head. No structural damage to the brain is caused, yet following concussion a person may suffer from headache, impaired vision and partial loss of memory.

conditioned reflex a response to a stimulus which has become automatic as a result of training (conditioning).

cones   the cells in the RETINA of the eye that are able to detect color.

congenital disorders   disorders present from birth.

congestion   an accumulation of material, such as blood or tissue fluid, in a vessel, channel or cavity. It is usually a reaction to injury, inhalation of harmful substances, infection, or an abnormality in venous or lymphatic drainage.

conjunctiva   the membrane covering the outer surface of the EYE and the inner surface of the eyelid.

conjunctivitis   inflammation of the CONJUNCTIVA.

connective tissue   cells and fibers that serve as a binding, supporting and packing medium around organs and muscles within the body.

constipation   the inability to defecate, or difficulty in achieving regular DEFECATION, often characterized by abnormally hard or dry feces.

contact lens   a small lens for correcting defective vision that is worn in contact with the surface of the eye.

continuous ambulatory peritoneal dialysis (CAPD)   a form of dialysis used instead of a larger, static kidney machine. It is based on a treatment known as PERITONEAL DIALYSIS. In CAPD the patient can walk around normally because the CATHETER or tube through which the dialyzing fluid is injected remains in the body. Only the bag containing drained-out fluid needs to be changed regularly.

contraception, or birth control   the prevention of PREGNANCY. The means of achieving this include "natural" methods; methods of preventing the male SPERM from fertilizing the female egg; and ways of stopping the development of a fertilized egg. One natural method is the rhythm method, which involves abstaining from intercourse during the fertile time of the MENSTRUAL CYCLE. Two common artificial methods of contraception are the use of the sheath (condom), a thin sheath of plastic or rubber that fits over the erect penis and collects the ejaculated sperm, and the DIAPHRAGM. Another is the INTRAUTERINE DEVICE (IUD), a small piece of plastic introduced into the womb to prevent the implantation of a fertilized egg. The use of a spermicide with all artificial aids is recommended. This is a chemical (foam, jelly, or pessary) that kills sperm in the vagina.

The "PILL" is a chemical contraceptive, taken orally, containing synthetic preparations of the HORMONES ESTROGEN and PROGESTERONE, which suppress ovulation.

convulsion a violent muscular spasm producing temporary twisting and involuntary jerks of the body and limbs. A series of them is commonly called a fit or a seizure, and is usually followed by a short period of unconsciousness.

corn a (hard or soft) painful thickening (callus) of the skin on or between the toes. It is usually caused by pressure or friction from ill-fitting shoes.

cornea the tough, transparent outer covering at the front of the eye.

corneal graft (medical name, keratoplasty) a surgical operation on the eye in which part or the whole of a damaged cornea is replaced by a healthy one.

coronary arteries branching arteries that supply the heart muscle with blood; there are two of them.

coronary artery disease deterioration of the CORONARY ARTERIES, usually associated with ANGINA pectoris, ARTERIOSCLEROSIS or ATHEROSCLEROSIS; untreated it can lead to a HEART ATTACK.

coronary thrombosis the blockage of one of the coronary arteries by a blood clot (thrombus). It causes a HEART ATTACK, and may result from progressive CORONARY ARTERY DISEASE.

corpus callosum the tracts in the brain linking the two cerebral hemispheres; these tracts contain millions of nerve fibers.

corpus luteum a yellowish mass of cells that forms in an OVARY at the place from which an ovum has been released. It produces the HORMONES progesterone and estrogen and helps to maintain PREGNANCY.

corpuscle a small rounded structure, commonly a BLOOD CELL. Red corpuscles are called erythrocytes; white corpuscles are leukocytes.

cortex the outer layer of an organ, as of

the CEREBRUM (cerebral cortex) of the brain or an ADRENAL GLAND.

Corti, Alfonso (1822–1876)   an Italian anatomist who discovered the organ of the inner ear (the ORGAN OF CORTI) by which sound is perceived.

corticosteroids   HORMONES secreted by the cortex of the adrenal gland.

corticotropin   better known as ACTH.

cortisol   another name for HYDROCOR-TISONE.

cortisone   a synthetically manufactured hormone of the steroid group, used to treat ALLERGIES, GOUT, RHEUMATOID ARTHRITIS, and some adrenal disorders.

coryza   the medical term for a COLD.

cosmetic surgery   a form of PLASTIC SUR-GERY, performed to improve or alter a person's appearance.

cough   the expulsion of air under pressure from the back of the throat. Persistent coughing is a symptom of several disorders, including BRONCHITIS, CROUP, LARYN-GITIS, PERTUSSIS, PNEUMONIA and TUBER-CULOSIS.

CPR   *see* CARDIOPULMONARY RESUSCITA-TION.

crab louse   a parasite that infests the genital region in a type of PEDICULOSIS.

cramp   a condition in which one or more muscles contract involuntarily, causing spasms of pain and sometimes immobility.

cranial nerve   one of twelve pairs of nerves that arise from the BRAINSTEM.

cranium   the bony covering of the brain, the upper and largest part of the skull.

cretinism   a disorder that causes an infant to develop into a mentally retarded dwarf as a result of an underactive THYROID GLAND.

crib death, or cot death   another name for SIDS (sudden infant death syndrome).

Crick,   Francis   Harry   Compton (1916–   )   an English biophysicist who shared with two other scientists, WILKINS and WATSON, the 1962 Nobel Prize in physiology and medicine for his pioneering studies on DNA (deoxyribonucleic acid). Wilkins had discovered the double helix shape of the DNA molecule and, using this information, Crick and Watson were able to determine the molecular structure of DNA and build a complete and accurate model of the molecule.

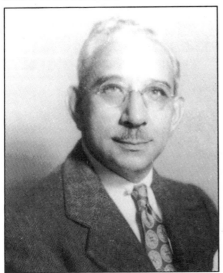

Crohn, Burrill B. (1884–1983) an American gastroenterologist who gained worldwide recognition for his description in 1932 of what is now known as Crohn's disease — a chronic inflammatory condition of the intestine.

cross-eye *see* SQUINT.

cross infection infection of one patient by another. This is a problem that occasionally occurs in hospitals.

croup an inflammation of the larynx, windpipe and bronchial tubes seen most commonly in infants and young children. Thick MUCUS is produced and there is a violent, rasping cough. The infection is usually caused by a virus but may sometimes be bacterial.

cryosurgery a surgical technique in which extreme cold is applied locally or generally to destroy unwanted tissue.

cryptorchidism is a condition in which a boy's testicles have failed to descend into the scrotum before birth.

Cushing, Harvey Williams (1869–1939) an American neurosurgeon who became renowned for his pioneering techniques in surgery on the brain and spinal cord. He was also the first to describe the symptoms of the rare adrenal disorder named CUSHING'S SYNDROME.

Cushing's syndrome   a group of symptoms resulting from overproduction of the hormone HYDROCORTISONE and other hormones from the adrenal glands. Among them are swelling of the face and neck, high blood pressure, acne, the wasting of muscles, obesity and excessive body hair. Such overproduction may be caused by a TUMOR (malignant or benign) affecting steroid secretion or the effects of steroid treatment.

cuticle   the epidermis, or thin outer layer, of the skin. It also describes a hard layer covering and protecting the epidermis, such as tooth enamel. In addition, it sometimes refers specifically to the dead skin occuring around the base of a fingernail or toenail.

cyanosis   a bluish coloration of the skin and lips that results from a lack of oxygen in the blood. A variety of disorders may be responsible for this condition, including lung disorders such as pneumonia.

cystic fibrosis   a noncontagious inherited disorder that commonly affects children up to adolescence. The EXOCRINE GLANDS become overactive and secrete abnormally thick MUCUS and sweat; these sticky secretions eventually interfere with the functions of the bile and pancreatic ducts, and the air passages, so that chronic lung disease and inadequate food absorption are characteristic. Although modern medicine has extended the average life span of afflicted individuals, no cure has been found and survival beyond young adulthood is rare.

cystitis   an inflammation of the bladder most often caused by bacterial infection. It is more common in women than in men, and may be acute or chronic; the major symptom is burning pain on urination.

cytoplasm   the protoplasm (structural and functional contents) of a cell, excluding the nucleus.

cytotoxic drugs   DRUGS used to destroy living cells. They are used particularly in CANCER treatment.

D

D and C (dilatation and curettage)   a minor operation in which the CERVIX is gently dilated or widened and tissue removed by scraping with a curette (an instrument shaped like a spoon).

dandruff   appears as small flakes of dead skin that lodge in the hair. It results from a condition of the SCALP in which the skin glands do not secrete enough moisture.

Darwin, Charles Robert (1809–1882) an English naturalist who gained worldwide fame with the publication in 1859 of *On the Origin of Species by Means of Natural Selection*. In this he produced evidence, much of it amassed while a naturalist aboard HMS *Beagle*, to support his theory that the process of evolution rested on natural selection.

deaf-mute   a person born completely deaf. A deaf-mute cannot speak, because he or she has never heard the sounds of speech and does not know what to imitate.

deafness   the partial or total inability to hear. Two main types are conductive deafness, in which sound cannot get through to the inner EAR; and perceptive or nerve deafness, in which the inner ear is damaged or incomplete.

death   the termination of life, which is medically accepted to have occurred when all activity of the brain ceases.

DeBakey, Michael (1908–)   a Texas surgeon who pioneered the manufacture and use of replacement arteries made from synthetic materials. He also invented a ventricular by-pass pump temporarily to sustain a heart weakened by surgery. These and other innovative techniques have placed him in the forefront of cardiovascular specialists.

debility   the medical term for physical weakness.

deciduous teeth   more commonly known as MILK TEETH.

decompression sickness, or the bends a disorder that results from over-rapid decompression after breathing air under pressure, as when deep-sea diving. Bubbles of nitrogen in the blood and tissues cause pain in the limbs. Gradual decompression prevents the disorder. If left untreated, however, serious problems may occur.

decongestants DRUGS used to treat certain respiratory disorders.

decubitus ulcer *see* BEDSORE.

defecation the action of releasing the FECES through the anus.

defibrillator a machine used to stop FIBRILLATION (jerky trembling of the heart muscle). The machine administers electric shocks which may restore the normal heartbeat. It can also stop and restart the heart for surgical purposes.

deficiency disorders are disorders that result from an inadequate diet or from an insufficient supply of VITAMINS or other essential metabolic factors. Among relatively common deficiency disorders are GOITER, RICKETS and iron-deficiency ANEMIA.

dehydration serious diminution of the water content in the body. It results either from abnormal loss of fluid or from decreased fluid intake. Symptoms include exhaustion. Treatment usually consists of small but frequent drinks of slightly salty water, and any measures practicable to correct the underlying problem. Untreated, severe dehydration may be fatal, particularly in infants.

Delgado, José a Spanish physiologist who, since the 1940s, has been experimenting with electrical stimulation of the brain. In experiments with monkeys and other animals, and using a remote control system, he has shown that he can successfully control the simple reactions in animal behavior. He envisages a time when human behavior could be similarly influenced.

delirium a serious mental disorder affecting the higher integrative functions, and characterized by agitation, hallucinations and confusion. There are many possible causes, including high fever, acute withdrawal from alcoholism, and toxins produced by bacteria.

delirium tremens a specific DELIRIUM associated with physical trembling and hallucinations, resulting from acute withdrawal from ALCOHOLISM.

delivery the birth of a baby, or parturition.

delusion   a false belief that is fairly held despite clear and compelling evidence to the contrary. It can be symptomatic of many medical and psychological disorders.

dementia   gradual mental deterioration caused by the degeneration and loss of brain cells. A condition that is relatively common in old age, it can also occur in ALCOHOLISM and SCHIZOPHRENIA.

dendrite   the fingerlike branch of a nerve cell body.

dental brace   a specific BRACE used in OR-THODONTICS to encourage the correct alignment of teeth.

dentin   a hard bonelike substance that makes up the major part of a tooth. It surrounds the pulp and is covered with an outer layer of enamel.

dentistry   the diagnosis and treatment — both curative and preventive — of disorders of the teeth, including the repair and replacement of damaged or lost teeth and the correction of the placement of teeth by means of ORTHODONTICS.

dentures   a set of false teeth. Sets of teeth are usually mounted on a metal brace or pegs, or fixed to a plastic plate.

deoxyribonucleic acid   *see* DNA.

dependence   the principal characteristic of ADDICTION to a drug; it is experienced both mentally and physically.

depilatory   any substance or device used to remove body hair. Alkaline creams are popular because they are painless and do not damage the hair roots. Electrolysis works by destroying the hair follicles with an electric current — and its effect is permanent.

depressants   DRUGS that reduce mental and physical activities and functions.

depression   in everyday terms means feeling blue or down. As a psychiatric term, major depression refers to a chemical imbalance commonly affecting sleep, appetite and mood.

dermatitis   inflammation of the skin.

dermatology   the study of the SKIN and its disorders.

dermatome   an area of skin supplied by

nerve fibers from a single spinal nerve. Also a surgical knife for cutting the skin.

dermis the innermost layer of SKIN. It contains nerves and nerve endings, sweat and sebaceous glands, blood vessels, and hair muscles and follicles.

densensitization a treatment for ALLERGY by overcoming an allergic person's sensitivity to the allergenic substances. This can be done by injecting the patient with increasingly strong doses of the substance until there is no further unfavorable reaction.

detached retina a condition in which the RETINA becomes separated wholly or in part from its supporting layer, the choroid. Symptoms include flashes of light and mistiness of vision. If untreated, the condition may develop into total blindness.

diabetes most commonly refers to diabetes mellitus, a disorder caused by lack of insulin in the body and characterized by excessive sugar in the blood and the urine. Symptoms include frequent urination, thirst, weight loss, and exhaustion. Untreated diabetics may lapse into a coma. Treatment may be through diet control or consist of oral hypoglycemic drug supplements or regular, balanced injections of insulin. Diabetes insipidus is characterized by excessive urination; it is caused by underproduction of VASOPRESSIN by the PITUITARY GLAND, or insensitivity of the kidney to vasopressin.

dialysis a way of artificially duplicating the natural functions of the kidney. The blood of patients suffering from kidney disease is passed into one compartment of a two-compartment tank separated by a special membrane. The membrane allows wastes to filter through to the second fluid, but retains useful larger particles such as proteins and blood cells. Pure blood is then returned to the patient's circulation.

diaper rash a red, inflamed area that appears on a baby's skin around the buttocks, thighs and genitals. It may be caused by badly laundered diapers (with insufficient rinsing), the ammonia content of the urine, or bacteria in the feces.

diaphragm the muscle located between the thorax and the abdomen, which contracts and relaxes during respiration. It is also a type of CONTRACEPTIVE device, also known as a Dutch cap, which is a rubber or plastic pessary that is fitted over the cervix to prevent sperm entering the womb.

diarrhea a condition marked by abnormally frequent defecation, voiding liquid feces before the water content has been fully absorbed by the colon. The resulting loss of fluid can lead to DEHYDRATION. It may be caused by various gastrointestinal disorders, including infection and poisoning.

diastole the relaxation of heart muscle, while the atria and ventricles fill with blood before SYSTOLE.

diet the type and quantity of food and drink habitually consumed by a person. It can also mean a choice regulated for medical treatment or to reduce or gain weight.

digestion the process by which food is broken down in the alimentary canal into simple substances that may be absorbed into the bloodstream.

digestive tract also called the alimentary canal or gastrointestinal system, the food canal from the mouth to the anus.

dilatation and curettage *see* D AND C.

diphtheria is a serious throat infection caused by a bacterium. Toxins secreted into the blood cause fever, a sore throat, and vomiting. Childhood immunization provides protection.

dipsomania *see* ALCOHOLISM.

disk commonly refers to the INTERVERTEBRAL DISK between two vertebrae in the SPINE.

dislocation usually the displacement of a bone from a joint; also of any organ from its normal position.

disorientation mental confusion in which the patient loses all awareness of identity, location and time. The condition may be caused by drugs, fever, poison or alcohol, or it may be a symptom of mental illness.

dissection most commonly refers to the cutting open of a dead body for scientific examination.

diuretics DRUGS that increase the output of urine from the kidneys in order to remove excess fluid from the body.

DIGESTION

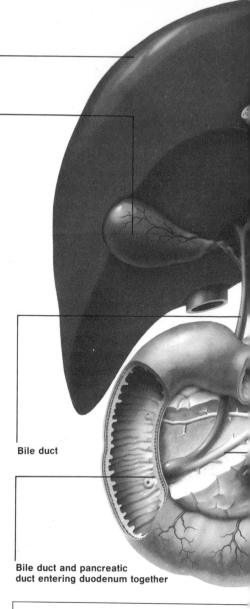

Liver

Gall bladder

Liver and pancreas are organs vital to the digestive process. The reddish-brown liver, weighing 3-4 pounds and divided into two lobes, is the largest internal organ. Bile is made in the liver and stored in the gall bladder until needed in the gut for the digestion of fats.

The pancreas is a pale red organ. It makes digestive enzymes which pass into the duodenum, the part of the intestine just below the stomach, via the pancreatic duct.

Bile duct

Bile duct and pancreatic duct entering duodenum together

The appendix is a finger-shaped bulge of gut near the junction of the small and large intestines. It is 3-5 inches long and hollow, and is larger in children than in adults. Its function is unknown, and digestion is not impaired if the organ is removed following the onset of appendicitis.

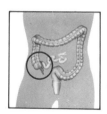

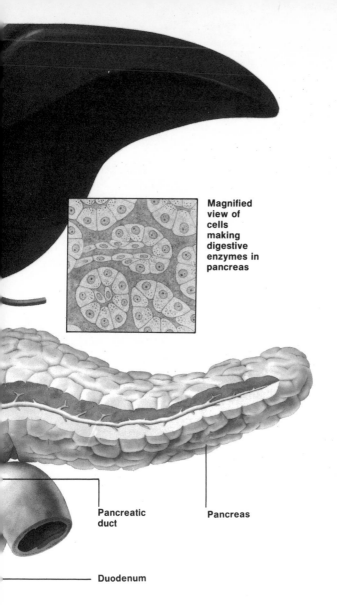

Magnified view of cells making digestive enzymes in pancreas

Pancreatic duct

Pancreas

Duodenum

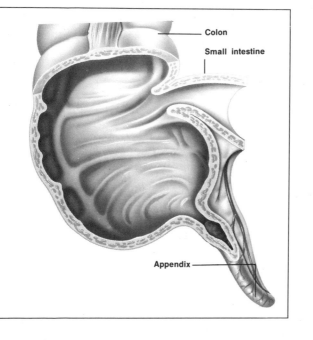

Colon

Small intestine

Appendix

59

diverticulitis inflammation of diverticula — pouches or sacs in the internal walls of the COLON. It usually results in pain, fever and constipation, and is treated with antibiotics and diet control.

dizziness a sensation of unsteadiness and lightheadedness.

DNA (deoxyribonucleic acid) a nucleic acid which is the basic component of GENES. A molecule of DNA may be represented as a double helix with two strands twisted around each other. It carries chemically coded messages that determine a person's HEREDITY.

dominant a term used in GENETICS to describe a GENE that is wholly or partly responsible for an identifiable characteristic in an individual.

dorsal on, near, or relating to the back of the body or an organ.

double vision (medical name, diplopia) seeing two images of a single object, one image with each eye. It may be the result of any of several eye disorders, including weakness or paralysis of one of the muscles that move the eyes. Intoxication by drugs or alcohol may also produce this symptom.

douche a stream of water or medical solution directed against some area of the body for hygienic or therapeutic purposes. It usually describes the internal washing of the female genitalia.

Down's syndrome, or trisomy 21 an inborn physical and mental condition formerly called mongolism. A person with this condition tends to have a short, squat body; a small head, widely-spaced eyes with a fold of skin at the inner corner; a flattish nose; and a high forehead. There is also noticeable mental retardation. The condition is caused by an extra CHROMOSOME, bringing the total up to 47 per cell instead of the normal 46. Affected persons have three of the twenty-first chromosome instead of two — hence the name trisomy 21.

DPT vaccine a combination of VACCINES used for immunizing infants. It is made up of DIPHTHERIA, PERTUSSIS (whooping cough) and TETANUS vaccines.

dreaming one form of mental activity during sleep, usually remembered as a series of imaginary visual events. RAPID EYE

MOVEMENTS (REM) occur beneath the closed eyelids during dreams, and there is changed electrical activity in the brain.

drip, or Iv the common name for an IN-FUSION of fluids through an INTRAVENOUS catheter, directly into the bloodstream.

drowning death by asphyxiation due to liquid in the airway.

drug addiction a specific type of ADDIC-TION.

drugs chemicals that have specific effects on part or all of the human body. They are classified according to the effects they have on the body. There are usually several different examples of drugs within each category.

drunkenness a state of intoxication by alcohol, which persists until the alcohol consumed is metabolized by the body.

Duchenne, Guillaume (1806–1875) a French physician who pioneered the use of electricity in the diagnosis and treatment of disease. One of the founders of neuropathology, Duchenne was the first to describe locomotor ataxia, progressive muscular paralysis, and the diaphragm's specific role in breathing.

duct any narrow canal or passage for secretions or fluids.

ductless glands glands that secrete HORMONES directly into the bloodstream; they are also known as ENDOCRINE GLANDS.

ductus arteriosus a blood vessel in a fetus that links the pulmonary artery with the aorta. This allows the blood supply to by-pass the lungs. It closes almost immediately after birth.

dumb without the ability to speak; it is another word for MUTE.

duodenal ulcer is an ULCER of the DUODENUM.

duodenum the first part of the small intestine, next to the stomach.

dura mater the outermost of the three layers of membrane called MENINGES which cover the brain and spinal cord. It is a tough, fibrous sheath.

dwarf an abnormally undersized person who may or may not be standardly proportioned. There are many possible causes of dwarfism, principal among which are hormonal abnormalities caused by deficiencies in PITUITARY secretion.

dysentery a disorder of the bowel, resulting from an infection that produces severe DIARRHEA containing blood and mucus. It is usually caused by bacteria or protozoa (such as AMEBA) absorbed from contaminated food or drinking water.

dyslexia, or word blindness a general term used to describe various disabilities in reading and writing. It varies from confusion between some letters to a complete inability to read.

dysmenorrhea difficult or painful menstruation. The causes may be psychological, or there may be a disorder of the womb or vagina. Painkilling and antispasmodic drugs may bring relief. Infection of the womb or vagina should be treated specifically with antibiotics.

dyspepsia indigestion involving vague abdominal pain (especially immediately after eating), heartburn and in some cases nausea and vomiting. Often made worse by emotional STRESS, these are a group of symptoms and not a disorder in themselves.

dyspnea *see* BREATHLESSNESS.

dystrophy the wasting away of tissue, or its failure to grow to normal strength. In the chronic condition known as MUSCULAR DYSTROPHY, a breakdown in muscle fibers causes weakness and degeneration in the muscles.

E

ear the sensory organ concerned with hearing, and associated with physical balance. It is made up of three parts. The external ear consists of the outer ear flap, or pinna, and the auditory canal, which ends at the eardrum. The middle ear, extending from the eardrum to the oval window of the cochlea, contains the three small bones known as auditory ossicles: the malleus, incus and stapes. The inner ear comprises the semicircular canals, concerned with the sense of balance, and the cochlea. Cells in the cochlea detect sound vibrations, providing us with hearing.

eardrum the thin membrane between the outer and middle ear.

earwax, or cerumen the WAX secretion produced by the lining of the external canal of the EAR.

eclampsia an uncommon condition that may occur during the last three months of PREGNANCY, in which the pregnant woman suffers high blood pressure, EDEMA, proteinuria and severe convulsions.

ECT *see* ELECTROCONVULSIVE THERAPY.

ectomorph a type of body shape, differentiated from ENDOMORPH and MESOMORPH. An ectomorph is, typically, tall and thin, with relatively little body fat.

ectopic pregnancy a dangerous condition of PREGNANCY in which a fertilized egg fails to reach the WOMB and implants itself instead in the FALLOPIAN TUBE. The EMBRYO may die and be absorbed or, after about two months' growth, it may rupture the Fallopian tube, causing hemorrhaging that may be life-threatening.

eczema a red, itchy inflammation of the skin. There are several different kinds of eczema; causes range from ALLERGY to irritation by household chemicals. None is contagious.

edema a swelling in any part of the body produced by an abnormal build-up of fluid in body cavities or tissues.

EEG *see* ELECTROENCEPHALOGRAPH.

egg another word for OVUM.

ego the conscious feeling, decision-making self of an individual. In PSYCHOANALYSIS, as defined first by Sigmund FREUD, it is distinguished from the primitive, instinctive ID and the civilized, self-conscious SUPEREGO as the primary site of memory, consciousness and awareness of reality.

Ehrlich, Paul (1854–1915) a German bacteriologist who pioneered the modern era of CHEMOTHERAPY, and coined the term itself. He searched all his life for a "magic bullet" against disease; shared the 1908 Nobel Prize in physiology and medicine for his work on immunization; and in 1910 announced a treatment for SYPHILIS, which was marketed under the trade name of Salvarsan.

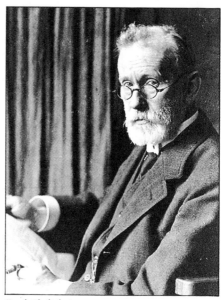

Paul Ehrlich (see previous page)

ejaculation an abrupt discharge of semen from the penis at the climax of sexual arousal in males.

EKG or **ECG** common abbreviation used for an ELECTROCARDIOGRAM.

elbow the joint in the ARM between the humerus bone of the upper arm and the radius and ulna bones of the forearm.

electrocardiogram (EKG) an electronically traced record of the electrical activity of the heart. It can be used as an aid in the diagnosis of heart disorders.

electroconvulsive therapy (ECT), or shock therapy an effective treatment for severe depression. A brief seizure is induced in an anesthetized patient by means of an electric current lasting a fraction of a second; the procedure replaces the former method of inducing a seizure by inhalation of insulin (insulin shock).

electroencephalograph (EEG) a machine for recording the electrical activity of the brain by means of electrodes placed on the scalp.

electrolysis the destruction of living tissue by passing an electric current through it. The method is commonly used as a DEPILATORY technique.

electron microscope a powerful microscope that uses a beam of atomic particles (electrons) projected onto a surface, instead of a beam of light through a lens, to produce a highly magnified image.

elephantiasis a disorder characterized by thickening and swelling of surface tissues of part of the body, usually the hands, legs, feet, or scrotum. The condition is usually caused by filarial worms that infest and block the lymph vessels that ordinarily drain these areas, so allowing fluid to accumulate in them.

emaciation the condition of being abnormally underweight.

embolism the blocking of a blood vessel by an air bubble, a foreign body, or a blood clot that has moved from its site of formation. Such a blockage may lead to a STROKE or to GANGRENE.

embryo the name given to an unborn baby from the moment of CONCEPTION to the end of the second month. After that it is generally called a FETUS.

emetic a substance which, when deliberately swallowed, causes vomiting.

emotion any strong feeling or mental disposition that arises subjectively and which produces certain physiological and psychological changes, particularly those affecting mood.

emphysema a chronic lung disorder in which the small air sacs in the lungs become abnormally enlarged as the intervening walls of tissue disintegrate. The major symptom is shortness of breath following any exertion.

enamel, dental the substance that covers the crown of a tooth. It is the hardest substance in the body.

encephalitis inflammation of the brain tissue, usually caused by a virus transmitted from ticks or mosquitoes. Bacteria or microorganisms can also cause the disease.

endemic disease a disease that persists in a certain place or among certain peoples. Continuously exposed, a population may thereby acquire a degree of immunity to the disease.

endocardium the mostly membranous inner surface of the cavities of the HEART, comprising endothelial, connective and muscular tissues.

endocrine glands secrete HORMONES directly into the bloodstream.

endocrinology the branch of science dealing with ENDOCRINE GLANDS and their secretions.

endocytosis a process in which the membrane of a CELL envelops and ingests a particle.

endometrium the lining of the WOMB, which changes during the MENSTRUAL CYCLE in response to the hormonal activity of the ovaries and the pituitary gland.

endomorph a type of body shape typified by a person who has round features and an abundance of body fat.

endorphin a type of chemical found in the brain that has tranquilizing and painkilling properties.

endoscope a pliable, usually fiberoptic, tube used for examining the inside of the body by being inserted through a natural orifice or a surgical incision.

endothelium the tissue made up of a single layer of cells which lines the heart, the lymph and blood vessels, and some other body cavities.

enema an introduction of fluid through the anus into the rectum and colon. It may be administered to flush out waste products or for a medical examination, usually by means of X ray.

energy the power and ability to do work. Fuel for the body's energy comes from food, which is broken down by the processes of digestion and absorbed by the body. Energy and heat are primarily manufactured in the body's cells; GLUCOSE, a simple sugar (from carbohydrates in food) is the main energy source. It is measured in CALORIES.

enkephalin a brain chemical similar in effect to an ENDORPHIN.

enzyme any of a number of protein substances produced by the body's cells which act as catalysts to control chemical changes within the body and speed up biological reactions. They are essential to life. Many enzymes, for instance, play a major part in digestion, breaking down specific foods to make them easily assimilable; only a minute trace may be needed to influence a reaction.

eosinophil   a type of white BLOOD CELL.

epicardium   the inner layer of the PERI-CARDIUM, the membrane that surrounds the HEART.

epidemic   an outbreak of a contagious disease that spreads widely and rapidly through a population.

epidermis   the outer layer of the SKIN.

epididymis   the long, narrow, tightly coiled tube in a male that connects the TESTICLE to the VAS DEFERENS.

epidural anesthetic   a local anesthetic injected into the space within the DURA MATER, the tough membrane that envelops the spinal cord. It is most commonly ad-ministered for pain relief during LABOR.

epiglottis   a leaf-shaped flap of fibrous cartilage behind the root of the tongue. During swallowing it covers the entrance to the LARYNX and so stops food from en-tering the TRACHEA.

epilepsy   a group of disorders in which there is abnormal electrical activity among the nerve cells of the brain. This activity recurs periodically and gives rise to con-vulsions. Symptoms range from GRAND MAL attacks, which involve unconscious-ness for up to several minutes with pro-nounced muscular spasms, to PETIT MAL att-acks, which may involve no more than momentary loss of consciousness.

epinephrine, or adrenaline   one of two HORMONES from the adrenal medulla, the other being NOREPINEPHRINE. Its main effects are to stimulate the heart, constrict the vessels of the peripheral circulation and relax the air passages in the lungs.

epitaxis   the medical name for a NOSE-BLEED.

epithelium   a layer of cells that covers most internal and external surfaces of the body. In some locations it produces mu-cous secretions and serves as a protection against infection and local tissue damage.

Epstein-Barr virus   a virus of the herpes family, which is the cause of GLANDULAR FEVER, or infectious mononucleosis, and Burkett's lymphoma.

equilibrium   *see* BALANCE.

erection   the enlarged and rigid state of the penis or the clitoris during sexual excitement, caused by mental or physical stimulation.

Erikson, Erik (1902–)   a German-born American psychoanalytical clinician who has explored the relationship between individual development and cultural environment. He studied the culture of American Indians and their ideas of bringing up children before publishing his classic textbook, *Childhood and Society*.

erysipelas   a painful skin infection caused by streptococcal bacteria. More commonly a disease in the elderly, it is marked by redness and swelling on the scalp, face or legs. It may be successfully treated with antibiotics.

erythema   an abnormal reddish discoloration of the skin caused by an increase of blood in the fine surface blood vessels. Sunburn and blushing are both examples of erythema.

erythroblastosis (fetalis)   *see* HEMOLYTIC DISEASE OF THE NEWBORN.

erythrocyte   a red BLOOD CELL.

erythrocyte sedimentation rate (ESR)   the rate at which red blood cells settle when an ANTICOAGULANT is added to the blood. An elevated rate indicates the existence of an inflammatory state.

esophagus   the gullet, the part of the alimentary tract between the mouth and the stomach.

ESR   *see*   ERYTHROCYTE SEDIMENTATION RATE.

estrogen   any one of a group of female sex HORMONES manufactured in the ovary and also in the adrenal lands. Estrogens affect the reproductive organs, and produce in women their distinctive female sexual characteristics.

ether   an organic chemical compound once widely used as a general anesthetic.

etiology   the cause of a disease, or more generally the study of the causes of disease. It is an important aspect of medical diagnosis.

eugenics   the science of the genetic improvement of species.

eunuch a male who has had his testicles removed.

euphoria a feeling of exalted jubilation and self-satisfaction. It may be a sign of mental disorder, although certain drugs may induce it artificially.

Eustachian tube the channel that connects the middle ear to the pharynx at the back of the throat.

euthanasia, or "mercy killing" the act of causing or enabling a person to die painlessly for compassionate reasons.

evolution the gradual anatomical change of organisms over a period of time, so that later species differ physically from their ancestors.

exanthem the medical name for a RASH that occurs as a symptom of a viral or bacterial infection.

excretion the elimination of wastes from the body, principally in the form of FECES or URINE. Exhaled air and sweating also remove waste products of the body's metabolism, mostly carbon dioxide and urea.

exercise any activity carried out to develop the muscles of the body, to train or keep fit. Exercise of the correct type improves muscle tone and stimulates the heart to pump blood more efficiently. There are many different types of exercises, including AEROBICS, calisthenics, gymnastics and JOGGING.

exhalation the respiratory action of breathing out.

exhibitionism in psychiatry, an overwhelming desire to attract attention to oneself by exaggerated or offensively inappropriate behavior.

exocrine gland a gland that secretes fluid to a target zone through a duct or tube, as is the case with the sweat glands or salivary glands.

exocytosis a process in which material from the CYTOPLASM of a CELL is enveloped by the cell membrane and expelled.

exophthalmos abnormal protrusion of the eyeballs. It is usually caused by overactivity of the thyroid gland, in exophthalmic GOITER.

expectorants DRUGS that encourage the expulsion by coughing of mucous secretions from the respiratory tract, particularly from the BRONCHIOLES.

extension the action of straightening a limb at a joint. It also describes the application of traction to a limb that has been fractured in order to ensure that broken bones knit and mend correctly.

extensor a muscle that moves bones away from each other around the fulcrum of a joint, thereby extending the limb, in contrast to a FLEXOR, which flexes a limb.

extracellular fluid all the fluid in the body not enclosed within the cells.

extra-uterine pregnancy *see* ECTOPIC PREGNANCY.

extrovert a term used in PSYCHOLOGY to describe a person who is generally more interested in external events than in inner feelings.

exudate any fluid that oozes out of the body, such as sweat, PUS or nasal MUCUS.

eye the organ of sight. Its chief parts include the curved, transparent CORNEA at the front which, together with the internal LENS, focuses light rays onto the RETINA at the back of the eyeball.

eyeglasses, or spectacles a pair of lenses housed in frames, which are worn in front of the eyes to correct sight defects. Such defects include ASTIGMATISM, HYPEROPIA and PRESBYOPIA. CONTACT LENSES are an alternative to conventional eyeglasses.

eyelash one of many short, curved hairs that fringe the eyelid as a protection for the eye against dust or other irritants.

F

face lift an operation to rejuvenate the appearance of the face by tautening the skin. It is an aspect of cosmetic or PLASTIC SURGERY.

Fahrenheit a scale of temperature devised by a German physicist of that name, and used for medical reference in many countries of the world. On this scale, 0° is the freezing point of a specific mixture of ice, salt and water; 32° is the melting point of ice (pure water); and 212° is the boiling point of water. "Normal" human body temperature is taken to be 98.6°F, although it varies from person to person.

fainting a sudden loss of consciousness caused by interrupted or inadequate flow of blood to the brain. It is called syncope, medically, but is commonly known as a blackout.

faith healing a process in which a sick person is cured through belief in the healing power of a faith healer.

Fallopian tube one of two channels, also called an oviduct, each of which connect a woman's OVARY to the top of the WOMB. Once a month, during childbearing years, one or other conveys an egg from an ovary to the womb.

Fallot's tetralogy a combination of four separate but related congenital heart defects: a hole in the partition between the ventricles ("hole in the heart"); blood reaches the aorta from both ventricles; the artery leading to the lungs is narrowed; and the muscle of the right ventricle becomes abnormally thickened. Symptoms are breathlessness and a bluish tinge to the skin; treatment is through corrective surgery.

false pregnancy (medical name, pseudocyesis) an emotional disorder in which a woman who is not pregnant displays most of the physical signs that she is.

false teeth *see* DENTURES.

family planning, or planned parenthood may be effected by various means. They include the RHYTHM METHOD for regulating sexual intercourse, and various methods of CONTRACEPTION.

fat a type of food in solid or liquid form that is a rich source of energy in the body, usually in ADIPOSE tissue.

fatigue a feeling of physical and mental tiredness, usually with an obvious cause, notably strenuous activity. It may also accompany convalescence after an illness. In certain cases, however, it is a symptom of a disorder or a disease, such as a nutritional deficiency, heart disease, certain infections, or psychological disturbances.

fatty acid one of a common series of organic acids, a number of which are formed as breakdown products of fats during the digestive process.

fatty tissue body tissue that contains naturally occurring fats.

feces, also known medically as stools the semi-solid waste products of digestion excreted through the anus. Their color, consistency and composition may provide a valuable diagnostic tool.

feedback mechanism the means in the body of self-regulation of internal processes; constant self-measurement of each process determines how much control over that process — often by glandular secretion — has to be effected. Many hormone levels, for example, are regulated by feedback mechanisms.

femur the anatomical name for the thighbone.

fertility the ability to have children. It depends on many factors, including hormone secretions, viable eggs and sperm, and correctly formed sexual organs.

fertilization, or conception the union of a sperm cell with an egg cell (ovum), which usually takes place in the upper part of a woman's FALLOPIAN TUBE. The single cell thus produced then multiplies, becomes implanted in the WOMB, and develops into an EMBRYO.

fetus the name given to an unborn baby from the beginning of the third month of pregnancy until birth. Before the third month it is usually called an EMBRYO.

fever an abnormally high body temperature that is more than 98.6°F as measured by an oral thermometer.

fever sore another name for a COLD-SORE.

fiberoptics the use of very fine long, transparent fibers in a flexible column to transmit an image via internal reflection. In medicine, a principal use is in an ENDOSCOPE.

fibrillation rapid and uncoordinated contractions of the HEART muscle, resulting in an irregular pulse.

fibrin an elastic, insoluble fibrous protein formed by the action of thrombin on the blood PLASMA protein fibrinogen. It causes blood CLOTTING by trapping blood

CELLS in its tangled threads.

fibrinogen a soluble protein present in the blood PLASMA. By the action of the enzyme thrombin it is converted into an insoluble protein, FIBRIN, which by creating a network of threads is essential for the CLOTTING of the blood.

fibroid a common but benign TUMOR that forms in the muscular wall of the WOMB. Larger fibroids may cause menstrual problems or exert pressure on other organs; otherwise, symptoms are rare.

fibula the smaller of the two bones of the lower leg, the other being the tibia or shinbone.

filament any fine, threadlike structure, such as the tail of a spermatozoon (male reproductive cell).

filtration the act or process of filtering. The kidneys filter waste products out of the blood, for example.

fimbria one of the fingerlike projections in the "fringe" at the opening of the FALLOPIAN TUBE, just below each ovary.

finger describes four out of five digits of each hand. Each finger is made up of three bones, called phalanges. The thumb — the fifth digit — has only two.

first aid emergency treatment given to sick or injured people before they can be conveyed to more institutional medical care.

fissure a groove or crack in a tissue.

fistula an abnormal hole or passage between a hollow organ and the body surface or between one hollow organ and another. It may be present at birth or develop from an ABSCESS or a surgical scar.

fit a common word for a seizure or CONVULSION. The word is also used in the context of good health, of "being fit."

flatfoot abnormal flatness of the sole and arch of the foot. The condition may be hereditary, or the result of an injury, or of being overweight.

flatulence an accumulation of gas in the stomach or intestines, accompanied by an urgent need to expel it. It may be produced by swallowed air or by the digestive processes.

flea one of a number of small, wingless, jumping, bloodsucking insects, belonging to the order Siphonaptera, which live as parasites on warm-blooded animals, including humans. Fleas may be vectors (carriers) of disease.

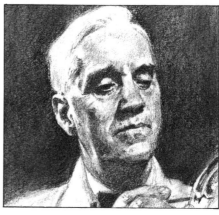

Fleming, Alexander (1881–1955) a Scottish bacteriologist. He discovered the antibiotic PENICILLIN by accident while working on bacteria-killing microbes. German chemist Ernst Chain and Australian pathologist Howard Florey isolated penicillin in 1940, and production was underway three years later.

flexion the action of bending a limb at a joint, or the condition of its being bent; the opposite — straightening — is extension.

flexor a muscle that causes FLEXION of a joint.

floating ribs the two lowest ribs (eleventh and twelfth), which do not join the breastbone (sternum).

flu *see* INFLUENZA.

flukes parasitic flatworms, several species of which may infest humans, attacking the intestine, lungs, liver or blood vessels.

fluoride a compound of the chemical element fluorine, found naturally in the soil and in some water. It helps to form bones and teeth, and thus to prevent teeth from decay.

fluoroscope an electronic device used in the diagnosis and study of the movements of the internal organs of the body. X-RAY pictures of the moving patient are presented virtually simultaneously on a video screen, thus avoiding the need for taking and developing single X-ray photographs.

focus   a point to which light rays converge or from which they appear to diverge, generally through the agency of a lens.

focusing, in vision   the act of altering the shape of the lens of the EYE so that light rays fall precisely on the retina to provide a clear image. It is also called ACCOMMODATION.

folic acid   a VITAMIN of the B complex that is necessary for the correct formation of red blood cells. It is found in green vegetables and meat.

folk medicine   the loosely defined body of popular treatments applied, with varying degrees of success, in communities in which orthodox practice is unavailable or regarded with suspicion.

follicle   a tiny cavity or sac, or a small, round, secretory gland of a type that occurs in many parts of the body. Each hair starts its growth from a hair follicle.

follicle-stimulating hormone (FSH)   a hormone produced from puberty in women by the pituitary gland. During each MENSTRUAL CYCLE it stimulates the growth of an ovarian or Graafian follicle, which ruptures to release an egg at ovulation.

fontanelle   is one of the six spaces that separate the eight skull bones of a newborn baby. The largest fontanelle is sometimes called the "soft spot." The bones, at first held together by a flexible membrane, fuse and become rigid after about eighteen months.

food poisoning   a general term describing acute gastrointestinal illness resulting from eating contaminated or poisonous food. Symptoms include stomach pain, vomiting and diarrhea.

foot   the lower end of the leg, which takes most of the weight of the body. It is made up of 26 bones and 33 joints.

forceps   pincerlike instruments used for grasping or extracting by surgeons and dentists. In CHILDBIRTH, a baby whose passage through the birth canal is restricted, may be delivered with the aid of forceps in what is called a forceps delivery.

forebrain   the front part of the brain, which develops into the CEREBRUM.

foreskin (medical name, prepuce)   the

formula

skin over the tip of the penis. It may be removed in the operation called CIRCUM-CISION.

formula in its popular sense, the mixture given to babies during BOTTLE-FEEDING.

fovea a small depression in a bone or other organ. It commonly refers to a depression on the retina of the eye.

fracture a break, particularly in a bone. There are five main ways in which bones can fracture: straight, from side to side; oblique or angled; twisted; splintered (comminuted); and greenstick, in which the bone splits to about halfway through and bends but does not break entirely. Other classifications are: simple, in which the skin is not broken; compound, if there is a surface wound; complicated, if internal organs are damaged; incomplete, when the bone is cracked but not completely broken; and depressed, if a flat bone (such as one in the skull) is dented and pushed inward.

fraternal twins, or non-identical twins TWINS born after two eggs are fertilized simultaneously.

freckles harmless brown marks that appear on the skin, usually after exposure to strong sunlight. They mostly occur on the face, backs of the hands and arms of people with a fair complexion. They are caused by accumulations of the dark pigment melanin in the epidermis of the skin.

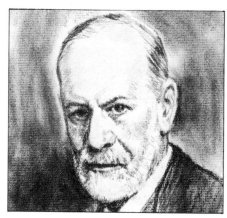

Freud, Sigmund (1856–1939) a Viennese neurologist and founder of PSYCHO-ANALYSIS. He believed that abnormal mental states such as hysteria could be traced to a complex of repressed and forgotten impressions. He claimed that sexual desires begin in infancy, and that dreams are an unconscious representation of such desires.

frigidity the persistent failure by a woman to enjoy or to reach a climax in sexual desire to enjoy sexual intercourse. The reasons are nearly always psychological, possibly involving feelings of guilt or abhorrence, or fear of pregnancy. Occasionally there may be a physical abnormality. It may be similar in cause to male IMPOTENCE.

frostbite damage to the skin and the underlying tissues caused by prolonged exposure to severe cold. Ears, nose, hands, and feet are the areas most likely to suffer frostbite.

frozen shoulder pain and stiffness in the shoulder. The direct cause is inflammation of the joint capsule, which may result from a strain. Because of the pain, the patient moves the shoulder infrequently. As a result, it may eventually "freeze" up altogether. Treatment is usually by physiotherapy and supervised exercises.

FSH *see* FOLLICLE-STIMULATING HORMONE.

fumigation the disinfecting of an area or clothing with gas fumes which are poisonous to germs and vermin (and often also to humans).

functional disorder, or inorganic disorder a disorder in which the function or activity of an organ is affected without any anatomical or structural cause or change. By contrast, organic disorders display physical changes in the structure of an organ or tissue.

fungus one of a group of organisms that include mushrooms, molds, and yeasts. Some are poisonous to humans if eaten; others, such as *Penicillium* (from which penicillin is derived), are helpful. Most fungal infections, such as ATHLETE'S FOOT, CANDIDIASIS, RINGWORM and THRUSH, affect the skin or mucous membranes.

furuncle another name for a BOIL.

G

Galen, Claudius (*c.* A.D. 125 – 200) a Greek writer and practitioner of medicine in Imperial Rome, renowned in his lifetime and famous, through his writings, for more than a thousand years afterward. Throughout Europe in the Middle Ages, he was regarded as the foremost authority in matters of medicine and health, especially in questions of human physiology.

gall bladder a small pouch or sac that lies beneath the liver and stores BILE until it is released into the DUODENUM, where it aids the digestion of fats. Inflammation of the gall bladder is called CHOLECYSTITIS.

gallstone a CALCULUS in the GALL BLADDER.

gamete a mature reproductive cell, a sperm or egg.

gamma globulin a GLOBULIN protein in the blood, which plays an important role in the IMMUNE SYSTEM.

ganglion part of the nervous system that may be described as a neutral "relay station" located outside the brain or spinal cord. The term is also technically used for a small, benign lump containing fluid that forms under the skin on the tendons.

gangrene the death and eventual decay of tissue caused by a failure of the local blood supply.

gastric juices the digestive acid secretions from the glands of the stomach. Hydrochloric acid and the enzyme pepsin are the principal gastric secretions.

gastric ulcer an ULCER of the stomach, also called a peptic ulcer.

gastroenteritis inflammation of the lining of the stomach and intestines, with symptoms and causes similar to FOOD POISONING.

gene a unit of heredity, located on a CHROMOSOME. Each gene is individually or in combination responsible for specific mental and physical characteristics inherited by a person. The essential chemical in the composition of a gene is DNA.

genetic drugs DRUGS identified by their pharmaceutical rather than their trade names.

genetic counseling a program of information and advice about human GENETICS provided for those planning parenthood. The counselor explains the influence of GENES and the kinds of genetic abnormalities that may occur, and goes on to assess the statistical chances of having an abnormal (genetically defective) child.

genetics the study of the principles of HEREDITY. Observation of inherited characteristics led scientists to postulate the existence of GENES, which carry genetic information. Microbiological techniques now enable genes not only to be identified individually, but also to be modified or repaired, which is the basis of genetic engineering.

genetic traits characteristics passed on from parents to offspring. Every person inherits pairs of GENES — one from the father and one from the mother — for each particular trait. In each pair the presence of a DOMINANT gene prevails in effect over any RECESSIVE gene also present.

genitalia the male and female reproductive organs, particularly the external sex organs.

genitourinary system those parts of the body concerned with the genital and urinary processes. It comprises the KIDNEYS, the URETERS, the URINARY BLADDER, the URETHRA and the associated reproductive organs.

geriatric of or pertaining to the elderly, with particular reference to diseases and disorders that affect them.

germ the common term for a microorganism capable of causing disease, known scientifically as a pathogen. It is also used to describe primitive living matter (a seed or a bud, for example) that can develop into an organism or organ.

German measles *see* RUBELLA.

gerontology the general study of aging.

gestation the period of pregnancy between CONCEPTION and CHILDBIRTH. In women, the gestation period is approximately nine months, or 280 days.

gigantism excessive growth during childhood and adolescence, resulting in an abnormal increase in height. The usual cause is overproduction of GROWTH HORMONE.

gingivitis inflammation of the GUMS, with painful swelling and bleeding as the gums begin to draw away from the teeth. Poor dental hygiene is usually the cause.

gland a structure of specialized cells that secrete fluids either directly into the blood (ENDOCRINE GLAND) or through a duct (EXO-

CRINE GLAND). The human body has more than 100 types of glands.

glandular fever (medical name, infectious mononucleosis)   a contagious viral disease. There is a marked increase in the number of certain white blood cells, and symptoms include enlarged lymph nodes, fatigue, headache and sore throat.

glaucoma   a group of painful eye disorders involving raised pressure in the fluid inside the eye. The condition is brought about by a narrowing or blocking of the narrow channel that carries fluid away from the eye into the veins. Symptoms include a hard, red eyeball and vision defects. Prompt treatment through drugs or, if necessary, surgery is needed to prevent blindness.

glia, or NEUROGLIA   cells that support nerve cells in the brain and spinal cord.

globulin   any of a group of proteins that occur in the blood. Globulins are classified as alpha, beta, or gamma globulins, according to their chemical behavior. Gamma globulins are ANTIBODIES; they play an important role in the body's IMMUNE SYSTEM.

glomeruli   small knots of capillaries located in the kidneys, inside the "cup" of a BOWMAN'S CAPSULE. They are the site of initial filtration of the blood in the kidneys.

glomerulonephritis   inflammation of the glomeruli, the minute collections of vessels that filter blood in the kidneys.

glossitis   inflammation of the tongue, which becomes sore and dark red; saliva turns sticky and thick, and there may be bad breath. It may be a symptom of anemia, gingivitis or septic teeth.

glottis   the site of sound-production in the LARYNX, between the two VOCAL CORDS.

glucocorticoid hormone   any of a group of adrenal cortical hormones (from the outer layers of the adrenal glands) which affect the metabolism of carbohydrates in the body.

glucose   a simple sugar, essential for energy, that occurs in the blood. It is a product of the breakdown of carbohydrates in food, or may be produced in the liver from GLYCOGEN.

glucose tolerance test   a test carried out

to see if a person is using and storing glucose normally, most commonly as part of the procedure for diagnosing DIABETES mellitus. The patient drinks a solution of about two ounces of glucose, after which blood samples are taken at regular intervals for two to five hours. The physician then looks for a persistently high blood sugar level.

glycemia   the presence of sugar or glucose in the blood. Hyperglycemia is excess glucose; hypoglycemia is too little glucose.

glycogen   a chemical formed in the liver and muscles from sugars and starches. It is the form in which GLUCOSE is stored, later to supply energy.

goiter   a swelling of the THYROID gland in the neck. It is usually caused by a lack of IODINE in the diet.

gonad   a sex gland; in a female the gonads are the two ovaries, in a male they are the two testes. Both originate from the same undifferentiated gonad in the embryo.

gonadotropin   a hormone secreted by the pituitary gland, which stimulates the GONADS.

gonorrhea   a highly contagious SEXUALLY TRANSMITTED DISEASE that attacks both men and women. Inflammation is accompanied by a yellow discharge from penis or vagina, though much less in women.

gout   a painful inflammation of the joints, caused by the kidneys failing to excrete excess uric acid so that crystals of it accumulate in the joints. It often begins with pain and swelling in the big toe.

graft   an organ or a piece of tissue transplanted to a part of the body in need of it. The healthy part may be taken from another person (the donor) or from the patient's own body (AUTOGRAFT).

grand mal   the more serious type of seizure that occurs in EPILEPSY.

granulocyte   a type of white BLOOD CELL.

gray matter   nerve tissue of the brain and spinal cord. It is brownish gray and is made up of nerve-cell bodies, threadlike extensions of the nerve-cell body called dendrites, and axons without the fatty substance myelin. Axons with myelin form the WHITE MATTER in the brain and spinal cord.

greenstick fracture   a type of FRACTURE in which a bone splits but does not break completely; it is particularly likely to occur in children.

grippe   *see* INFLUENZA.

gristle   *see* CARTILAGE.

groin   the region of the front of the body where the muscles of the legs join the abdomen. It is also called the inguinal region.

group therapy   a method of psychiatric treatment for people with NEUROSIS or other mental problems. Small groups meet together at regular intervals, under the passive guidance of a psychotherapist, and talk freely about their own and each other's problems.

growth   development and increase in size. Factors affecting human growth include heredity (the height and weight of the parents), living conditions, diet, disease, and the secretion of certain hormones, particularly GROWTH HORMONE.

growth hormone   a HORMONE (also called somatotropin) produced by the front part of the pituitary gland. It stimulates growth of the bones — particularly long bones — and other tissues.

gullet   a common term for the ESOPHAGUS.

gums   structures made up of connective tissue which cover the jawbones and contain the tooth sockets. The gums also envelop the bases of the teeth.

gut   another word for the INTESTINES, sometimes also used to include the STOMACH and ESOPHAGUS.

gynecological disorders   disorders that affect the reproductive organs of women.

gynecomastia   the overdevelopment of one or both breasts in a male, usually the result of HORMONE imbalance and most likely to occur temporarily at PUBERTY.

H

habit   an addiction, or a constant tendency to perform an act.

habituation   the process of forming a HABIT, but particularly becoming addicted to a drug such as alcohol.

hair   a thin, tubular structure of usually pigmented dead cells composed of the protein keratin. It has a hollow core and grows from a HAIR FOLLICLE.

hair follicle   a pit in the skin that produces a hair. The root of the hair is embedded in the bottom of the follicle, which is well supplied with blood vessels. The hair grows because of a group of cells at the base which constantly divide and multiply.

Haldane, John Burdon Sanderson (1892–1964) a British mathematician and scientist who was best known for his mathematical study of population GENETICS. He also did valuable work in physiology, and discovered the similarities between the inheritance of HEMOPHILIA and COLOR BLINDNESS.

Hales, Stephen (1677–1761)   an English physiologist and pastor who conducted early studies on blood movement, arterial pressure in humans and plant transpiration.

halitosis   bad breath. The cause may be tooth decay, infection of parts of the nose, mouth and throat, poor oral hygiene, or disorders of the stomach and intestine.

hallucination   the perception of something that is not physically present. Although most commonly visual, it may involve any of the five senses.

hallucinogens   DRUGS that produce hallucinations.

hallux valgus   the angulation of the great, or big, toe away from the midline of the body, toward or across the other toes.

hammertoe, also called claw toe   a deformity of the bones of the toe in which the first joint is bent downward to produce a clawlike shape.

hamstring   one of a group of TENDONS connected to muscles at the back of the knee. The muscles are also known as hamstrings.

hand

hand the lower end of the human arm, below the wrist. The framework of the palm comprises CARPAL (wrist) and META-CARPAL bones. The four fingers of the hand each have three PHALANGES; the thumb has two.

handicap any physical or mental disability that interferes with a person's normal activities.

hangover a popular term for the symptoms that follow the drinking of too much ALCOHOL. These include headache, nausea, thirst and dizziness.

Hansen's disease *see* LEPROSY.

Harary, Isaac an American biochemist who discovered that most young heart cells had the potential to beat spontaneously. He found that certain muscle cells initiate an electric impulse that is imparted to touching, hitherto non-beating cells. He called these cells "leading" cells, and surmised that most of them lay in the heart's pacemaker region.

hardening of the arteries describes the condition ARTERIOSCLEROSIS.

harelip a defect present from birth which takes the form of a cleft in the front of the upper lip. It is caused by the failure of parts of the facial tissues of the fetus to unite. It is often associated with CLEFT PALATE.

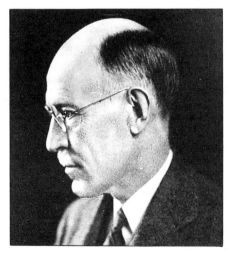

Harrison, Ross (1870–1959) an American biologist who pioneered the technique of tissue culturing. He devised the method in order to observe nerve fibers growing. He produced the first successful tissue culture in 1907, and this made it possible for the first time to observe, grow, and experiment on living cells outside their normal environment.

Harvey, William (1578–1657) an English physician and anatomist who discovered the circulation of the blood. Harvey experimented for twelve years with more than 80 species of animals before publishing his *An Anatomical Essay on the Motion of the Heart* in 1628. It contradicted GALEN's 1,500-year-old dogma about the function of the heart and revealed the blood's one-way path.

Haversian system any one of many cylindrical units that make up the hard compact shell of bones. Each unit forms a minute canal for an artery, vein, and lymph vessel.

hay fever a condition brought on by an allergy to one or more species of pollen. Symptoms are nasal irritation, sneezing, and a running and stuffy nose. Antihistamine and anti-allergic DRUGS may bring relief.

headache a common complaint which, though painful, is usually fairly harmless; an unexplained headache may, however, be a symptom of a serious disorder.

hearing the proprioceptive sense associated with the EAR.

hearing aid a small electronic apparatus worn inside or just behind the ear to help people with varying degrees of DEAFNESS. It consists of a receiver, amplifier, and earpiece.

heart the muscular organ in the chest which pumps blood throughout the body.

heart attack (known medically as a myocardial infarction) an acute condition of pain in the chest and shortness of breath produced by a CORONARY THROMBOSIS. It occurs when a clot blocks one of the arteries supplying blood to the heart muscle. A heart attack may stop the heart completely, causing death, although with prompt treatment (such as CARDIOPULMONARY RESUSCITATION) the patient may survive.

heartbeat the regular rhythm caused by the pumping of the heart muscles. It can be readily detected by feeling the PULSE. A healthy adult rate is about 70 to 80 beats a minute while at rest.

heart block   a slowing down or lack of coordination in the beating of the heart. It is caused by damage to the fibers that carry the nerve impulses within the heart muscle.

heartburn   a colloquial term for INDIGESTION. It is caused by stomach acids flowing back into the sensitive ESOPHAGUS, which produces a burning feeling in the center of the chest.

heart disease   a general term used to describe a large number of disorders. They include CORONARY ARTERY DISEASE, FIBRILLATION, FALLOT'S TETRALOGY in the newborn, HEART ATTACK, HEART MURMUR and VALVULAR DISEASE OF THE HEART.

heart-lung machine   a machine that bypasses the heart and lungs while still maintaining the circulation of oxygenated blood round the body. It is used during heart surgery.

heart murmur   an abnormal sound produced by the heart. It is caused by an irregularity in the blood flow through the chambers and valves of the heart.

heart-pacemaker   either the natural PACEMAKER, known as the sino-atrial node, in the heart or an artificial stimulator which can be implanted to replace or reinforce this.

heart rate   the number of heartbeats per minute.

heart transplant   the replacement of a diseased HEART with a healthy one from a donor recently certified brain dead.

heart valve   one of four valves in the heart. As blood flows from the right atrium to the right ventricle it passes through the tricuspid valve; between the right ventricle and the pulmonary artery is the right semilunar (pulmonary) valve; between the left atrium and the left ventricle is the mitral valve; and between the left ventricle and the aorta is the left semilunar (aortic) valve.

heatstroke   a condition resulting from prolonged exposure to heat, particularly that of the sun. Symptoms are a high temperature, a flushed dry skin, vomiting, and perhaps loss of consciousness. Sunstroke is a form of heatstroke.

heavy metals   certain metallic elements — such as cadmium, mercury and lead — that are extremely poisonous to the human body, even in minute quantities.

heel the rear part of the foot; the heel bone is the calcaneus.

height many factors influence height: genetic factors are important but height is also affected by living conditions, food, hormones, disease and possibly even emotional factors. Most adolescents put on a GROWTH spurt in their early teens. People are usually tallest at around age 20. After that they begin to gradually and slightly shrink.

Heimlich maneuver an emergency technique for clearing the windpipe of a person who is choking.

hematemesis vomiting of blood. It may be the result of a nosebleed or a symptom of something much more serious, such as bleeding from a peptic ULCER. Acid in the stomach turns the blood very dark.

hematology the study of blood and disorders of the blood.

hematoma a blood clot that forms in an organ or in the tissues, usually as a result of injury or surgery. A BRUISE is a type of subcutaneous hematoma.

hematuria the presence of blood in the urine, which may be cloudy, pink, red or dark brown. It may be a symptom of a kidney disorder or of inflammation of the bladder.

hemiplegia paralysis affecting one side of the body only.

hemoglobin a red iron-based pigment contained in the RED BLOOD CELLS which combines readily but loosely with oxygen. These cells transport oxygen from the LUNGS to the tissues of the body.

hemolysis destruction of the red blood cells accompanied by the release of hemoglobin. The reduced number of red blood cells in the circulation may cause ANEMIA.

hemolytic disease of the newborn (HDN) a life-threatening condition affecting newborn babies. It arises from incompatibility between the blood type of the baby and that of the mother, often a rhesus incompatibility.

hemophilia a group of HEREDITARY blood diseases characterized by severe, sometimes spontaneous, bleeding in any part of the body, caused by the lack of any of several essential CLOTTING factors in the blood. The disorder is incurable.

hemorrhage bleeding, which may be external or internal.

hemorrhoids, or piles a painful and irritating condition of swollen veins in the rectum or anus. Experts believe that one contributing factor may be constipation caused by low-fiber diet.

heparin one of several anticoagulant DRUGS, which prevent blood CLOTTING.

hepatic portal vein collects blood from the vessels supplying the STOMACH, INTESTINES and SPLEEN, and conveys it to the LIVER, where hepatic filtration occurs before the blood returns to the circulation through the hepatic veins and the inferior VENA CAVA.

hepatitis inflammation of the liver. Commonly caused by infection with a virus, it may also be caused by chemicals or drugs. One of the typical symptoms is JAUNDICE.

heredity the natural phenomenon by which one living creature carries some of the characteristics, principally of a physical type, of its direct (or sexual) ancestors. The mechanisms of heredity are studied in GENETICS.

hermaphrodite a person possessing both male and female organs and sexual characteristics.

hernia, or rupture a lump or swelling resulting when an organ or mass of tissue breaches its supporting muscular wall. The most common type is an inguinal hernia, which occurs in the groin when part of the intestines push their way through weakened muscles of the groin. Others include a hiatus hernia and umbilical hernia, which sometimes affects newborn babies.

heroin a strong, painkilling addictive drug derived from the opium poppy.

herpes one of a number of virus diseases marked by irritating or painful blisters and other skin eruptions. *Herpes simplex* is the COLDSORE, and *Herpes zoster* is CHICKENPOX or SHINGLES. *Herpes genitalis* is a sexually-transmitted virus.

Hess, Walter Rudolph (1881–1973) a Swiss physiologist who in 1949 shared the Nobel Prize in physiology and medicine with the Portuguese neurologist Egas Moniz. He discovered that emotions could be electrically induced and controlled in certain mammals.

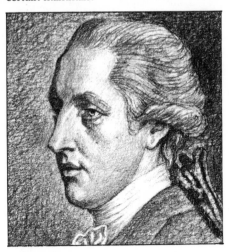

Hewson, William (1834–1869) an English anatomist who, through his researches into the nature of blood, became the first to realize that FIBRINOGEN, which he called "coagulable lymph," was the natural agent in the blood that caused clotting.

hiccup, or hiccough a spasmodic contraction of the DIAPHRAGM, which causes the sudden closure of the glottis (the vocal apparatus of the larynx) at the time of taking a breath. It may be caused by eating too fast, by swallowing a stomach irritant, or by local diaphragmatic irritation.

Hill, Archibald Vivian (1886–1977) a British biophysicist who shared the 1922 Nobel Prize in physiology and medicine for his discoveries in the physiology of muscle contraction.

hind brain the part of the brain nearest to the spinal cord. It consists of the MEDULLA OBLONGATA, the PONS and the CEREBELLUM.

hip the joint between the FEMUR of the leg and the PELVIS. The socket in the pelvis is the ACETABULUM or hip joint.

hippocampus part of the LIMBIC SYSTEM of the brain (which is associated with the emotions).

Hippocrates (*c.* 450–390 B.C.) a Greek physician and teacher renowned for the oath he formulated and required his students to take before practicing their skills. The oath is concerned principally with the ethics of practice of a physician,

HORMONES

Hypothalamus in brain

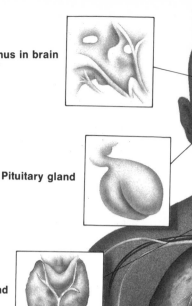

Pituitary gland

Thyroid gland

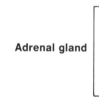

Adrenal gland

Pancreas

Testicles

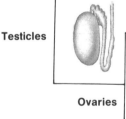

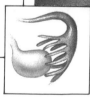

Ovaries

HORMONE PRODUCERS

Some of the many organs that produce and release hormones are shown to the left of the illustration. These hormones are chemical messengers, carried in the bloodstream, which ensure the coordinated functioning of many body organs.

The events shown on the ri[g] of the illustration happen automatically as a result of hormone activity in respons[e] danger. The signalling come[s] from the pituitary gland, jus[t] beneath the brain, which releases the hormone ACTH

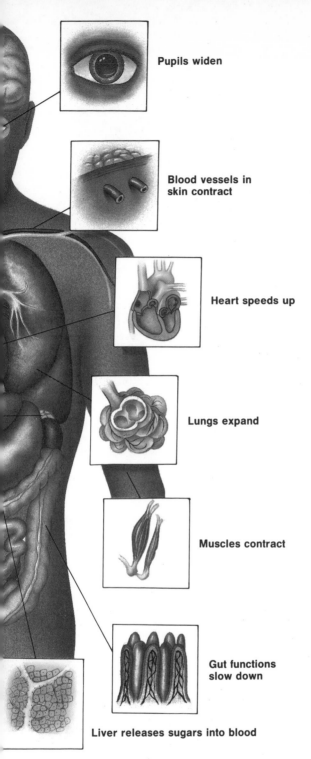

Pupils widen

Blood vessels in skin contract

Heart speeds up

Lungs expand

Muscles contract

Gut functions slow down

Liver releases sugars into blood

RESPONSES TO STRESS

the blood when danger
tens. When the hormone
es the adrenal glands on
f the kidneys it stimulates
to produce epinephrine
naline) and other
ating hormones.
response, the heart speeds

up, the lungs expand, the liver
releases sugars into the blood
for energy, and blood is
shunted to the muscles and
away from other organs.

and provides a sound ethical basis even today.

hirsutism a condition marked by excessive growth of hair, or hair growth in unusual places. The term usually describes a condition in women because their body hair growth is normally limited.

histamine a chemical present in most body tissues. It is released after any local damage, and is responsible for the characteristic symptoms of inflammation.

histiocyte a type of MACROPHAGE that occurs in some CONNECTIVE TISSUE.

histology the microscopic study of the tissues of animals and plants.

hives, or nettle rash (medical name, urticaria) a symptom of an ALLERGY. It is characterized by the eruption of weals on the skin resembling those produced by nettle stings.

Hodgkin, Alan (1914–), and **Huxley, Andrew** (1917–) two English biologists who were jointly awarded the Nobel Prize in physiology and medicine for 1963 for their pioneering work into the movements of ions in the excitement of the nerve membranes. Their highly important understanding of nerve impulse transmission was gained largely from experiments on the nerve fibers of squids and crabs.

Hodgkin's disease, or Hodgkin's lymphoma a disorder of the LYMPHATIC SYSTEM which results in enlarged lymph nodes and spleen, associated with swelling of the liver and other tissues. Its cause is not known.

holistic medicine a term denoting an approach to medical practice that tries to regard the body as a whole organism rather than concentrating exclusively on specific aspects or disorders. It also tries to be more open-minded than orthodox practice about the value of ALTERNATIVE MEDICINE.

homeopathy a form of ALTERNATIVE MEDICINE based on the theory of treating a disorder with small amounts of drugs which in a healthy person would produce identical symptoms if given in larger quantity.

homosexuality sexual attraction to (and possibly sexual relations with) persons of the same sex. Female homosexuals are commonly called LESBIANS.

hormone   a chemical produced by specialized tissues (ENDOCRINE GLANDS) in the body and secreted by them generally directly into the bloodstream from where they exert stimulatory or inhibitory effects on other body tissues.

hot flashes   sudden waves of heat that sometimes envelop the whole body, particularly as a symptom of the MENOPAUSE. They are generally caused by HORMONE imbalance.

housemaid's knee, or prepatellar BURSITIS   an inflammation of the bursa at the knee joint.

Hubel, David and **Wiesel, Torsten** two American neurobiologists who, since the late 1950s, have been investigating the brain's visual processing mechanisms. Their work won them a Nobel Prize in physiology and medicine in 1981.

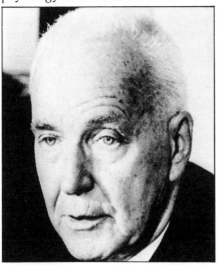

Huggins, Charles Brenton (1901–   ) a Canadian-born American physician who pioneered the treatment of cancer by CHEMOTHERAPY. In 1941, he began successfully to treat patients suffering from PROSTATE tumors with HORMONES. He shared the 1966 Nobel Prize in physiology and medicine.

humerus   the bone of the upper arm.

hunchback, or humpback (medical name, kyphosis)   curvature of the spine so severe that the back seems to have a hump in it. Causes may be congenital, an injury, or any of various diseases.

hunger   the feeling of distress, weakness,

Hunter, John

and urgency to eat caused by a lack of food.

Hunter, John (1728–1793)   an outstanding Scottish surgeon and anatomist who taught the revolutionary theory that the skeleton was made of complex living tissue, which was constantly renewing itself. He was one of the first to realize that the healing of bone fractures could be accelerated by movement and moderate pressure.

Huntington's chorea   a specific type of CHOREA in which mental disturbances occur in addition to the involuntary movements found in chorea. The disease is inherited exclusively by males, in whom symptoms appear between their thirties and their fifties. It is relentlessly progressive and there is no specific cure.

Huxley, Hugh (1924–   ) and **Huxley, Andrew** (1917–   )   two scientists who coincidentally share the same surname. They worked to evolve the same revolutionary theory at the same time, and independently declared that when a muscle as a whole contracts, the minute components of its individual fibers slide past each other but do not actually contract themselves.

hydatid cyst   a CYST that forms in an organ such as the liver, and encloses within it the eggs of a tapeworm, *Echinococcus*, that is parasitic in some wild and domestic animals and is contracted through contaminated meats.

hydrocephalus   a usually congenital disorder in which a baby's brain ventricles grow progressively larger because of CEREBROSPINAL FLUID trapped within them; in an infant the skull may eventually enlarge. Without surgery this condition can result in brain damage.

hydrocortisone, or cortisol   an important natural hormone secreted by the ADRENAL GLANDS. It regulates the action of glucose, fats and water in the body, and is used as a drug to treat ADDISON'S DISEASE, ASTHMA, rheumatoid arthritis and allergies.

hygiene   the study of health and the observance of rules of health and cleanliness. The latter is an essential part of preventive medicine.

hymen   the thin membrane just inside the vagina which partly or almost completely closes it. If not already broken, it is ruptured during a woman's first experience of sexual penetration.

hyoid bone   a U-shaped bone located at the base of the tongue, and at the top of the neck.

hyperactivity, or hyperkinesia   a condition in which a child appears to be overactive. It may be a symptom of a psychological, neurological or endocrine disorder.

hyperglycemia   a condition in which there is an abnormally high level of GLUCOSE in the blood. It is, for example, a result of DIABETES mellitus.

hyperopia, or farsightedness   a defect of vision in which close objects appear blurred whereas distant objects are seen clearly. Light rays tend to focus behind the retina either because the distance between lens and retina is too short as a result of heredity, or because of incapacity in the refractive power of the lens. The condition is regarded as a symptom of aging.

hypertension   the medical term for high BLOOD PRESSURE.

hyperthyroidism, or thyrotoxicosis   a condition in which the THYROID GLAND produces an abnormal amount of thyroid hormone. Insomnia, sweating and palpitation are some of the symptoms; treatment is predominantly by drugs.

hypertrophy   abnormal enlargement of body tissues in an organ. It may occur as the result of exercise, as with a limb muscle, or from disease. The heart muscle, for example, may enlarge following a period of high blood pressure.

hyperventilation, or overbreathing   an increase in the rate and depth of inhaling to more than normal.

hypnosis   a method to produce an artificial trancelike condition. The hypnotist induces this state in a susceptible subject by means of suggestion. Deep hypnosis is sometimes used to combat phobias and relieve pain.

hypochondria   a state of constant but (usually) groundless concern about one's own health and well-being.

hypodermic   beneath the skin; the term generally refers to the injection of a drug or vaccine administered by means of a syringe attached to a hollow needle. The term is also an abbreviation of the full name: hypodermic syringe.

hypoglycemia   a condition in which the GLUCOSE content of the blood is abnormally low.

hypophysis   the PITUITARY GLAND.

hypopituitarism   a condition in which there is diminished — and insufficient — secretion of the PITUITARY hormones, in adults leading to general debility, but in young children often leading to dwarfism unless treated.

hypothalamus   part of the brain between the THALAMUS and the PITUITARY GLAND. It helps regulate pituitary secretions and also coordinates activities of the SYMPATHETIC and PARASYMPATHETIC NERVOUS SYSTEMS.

hypothermia, or exposure   a condition in which the temperature of the body is abnormally low, usually following exposure to a cold environment. The very young and the very old are least able to resist it.

hypothyroidism   a condition produced by underactivity of the thyroid gland. If it occurs before birth, the baby is mentally and physically handicapped.

hysterectomy   the surgical removal of the uterus (WOMB).

hysterical conversion   loss of a physical ability — commonly hysterical paralysis or hysterical blindness — for psychological reasons.

I

iatrogenic disorder   any abnormal mental or physicial condition resulting from medical treatment.

icterus   another name for JAUNDICE.

id   in PSYCHOANALYSIS, the most primitive and instinctual of the three parts of the human mind. Its unconscious urges are modified by the other two parts, known as the self-conscious SUPEREGO and the mediating EGO.

identical twins, or maternal twins. TWINS born when one fertilized OVUM divides so that two genetically identical embryos develop. Non-identical twins are known as FRATERNAL TWINS.

ileum the lower part of the small intestine, linking the JEJUNUM to the CECUM. In it, the digestion of carbohydrates and fats is completed.

illusion a mistaken impression, usually visual, that occurs when the senses misinterpret the information they receive. Fever, drugs and alcohol may alter consciousness to make illusions more likely. It differs from a DELUSION in that the latter is a belief held in spite of all evidence to the contrary, and from HALLUCINATION in that the perception is not imagined although it is misinterpreted.

immune response a function of the body's defensive IMMUNE SYSTEM which protects against invading organisms. In response to the presence of ANTIGENS, the body produces neutralizing ANTIBODIES.

immune system the body's natural long-term defense system against invading disease organisms. It is based on the struggle between foreign bodies called ANTIGENS (viruses, bacteria, poisons, for example) and ANTIBODIES, proteins produced by the body in response to specific antigens.

immunoglobulin any protein in PLASMA that is capable of acting as an ANTIBODY.

immunosuppressives drugs used following surgery — especially TRANSPLANT SURGERY — to suppress the body's natural IMMUNE RESPONSE so that tissue grafted or donated has less chance of being rejected.

impacted wedged together so that movement or growth is impossible. A broken bone of which the jagged edges are forced together is said to be impacted.

impetigo a contagious skin disease caused by bacteria. It forms sores that are soon covered with thick yellow crusts. It is initially treated with antiseptic or antibiotic creams or lotions.

implantation the process by which a fertilized egg, after moving down the Fallopian tube and after dividing several times, embeds itself in the lining of the mother's uterus (WOMB).

impotence the inability of a man to experience an erection and thus successfully participate in sexual intercourse. It may have psychological or physical causes.

incisors the chisel-shaped TEETH at the front of the mouth.

incontinence   a condition involving a loss of control over the bladder or the muscles of the rectum and anus. As a result, a sufferer is unable to regulate urination or control bowel movements.

incubation period   the interval between exposure to infection and the appearance of the first symptoms. It may range from a few days — for example in the case of diphtheria — to as long as a year in some types of rabies. The period also determines the duration of QUARANTINE.

incubator   is an enclosed transparent box that provides a protective environment of warmth, humidity and oxygen appropriate for babies who have been born prematurely.

incus   one of the three tiny bones of the middle EAR. The other two are the malleus and the stapes.

indigestion (medical name, dyspepsia) the burning sensation under the breastbone commonly called HEARTBURN, felt after eating. The cause may be eating too much or too rich food, eating a large meal before going to bed, a disorder of the esophagus or stomach, or a psychosomatic problem.

induction of labor   the initiation or hastening of childbirth by artificial means. One method is by the injection of the hormone oxytocin to stimulate the contractions of the womb. Another is to surgically rupture the amniotic sac.

industrial diseases   illnesses contracted in the course of work, classified as OCCUPATIONAL DISORDERS.

infarction   the forming of an area of dead tissue (infarct), caused by a blockage in a blood vessel that has interrupted the blood supply to the area. The most significant infarcts occur in the brain, lungs, and heart.

infection   invasion of the body by harmful organisms (pathogens), such as viruses, bacteria, fungi and protozoans. Attack by parasites is commonly called infestation.

infectious mononucleosis   *see* GLANDULAR FEVER.

inferiority complex   the psychological term for a state of mind in which a person experiences a pervasive sense of inadequacy.

infertility   the inability to have children.

There are many possible causes, both anatomical and physiological. Infertility may even occur in a couple who are both potentially fertile, but are immunologically incompatible.

infestation   the harboring on or in the body of parasites such as fleas or worms.

inflammation   the natural reaction of tissue and blood vessels to injury or infection (or occasionally to the presence of an ALLERGEN). Increased amounts of blood and body fluids are released, partly under the influence of HISTAMINE, to the affected part to promote healing. The result is redness, pain, heat and swelling.

influenza, or flu   a highly contagious, sometimes EPIDEMIC, disease of the upper respiratory tract caused by a VIRUS. Symptoms resemble those of a severe COLD.

infrared radiation   invisible heat radiation with wavelengths beyond the red end of the visible spectrum. It is used by physiotherapists to relieve pain.

ingrowing toenail   a condition in which the front edge of a toenail grows into the soft tissue alongside and causes inflammation, often the result of poor foot hygiene or ill-fitting shoes.

inguinal hernia   a HERNIA in which part of the intestines are forced through the inguinal canal in the groin.

inhalant   a medicinal preparation for inhaling to relieve bronchial disorders such as ASTHMA.

inhalation   the act of drawing into the lungs. As a treatment it may involve breathing in a gas or vapor for therapeutic purposes.

inheritance   the sum total of all the characteristics derived by one generation from an earlier one by heredity.

inhibition   a specific area of diminished function caused by unconscious psychological conflict.

injection   the introduction of a fluid into the body, usually by means of a HYPODERMIC syringe.

inkblot test   common name for the Rorschach test, in which the subject verbalizes immediate associations with a standardized series of inkblots. The associations are used to assess personality and EGO functions.

inner ear contains the vestibular apparatus, the SEMICIRCULAR CANALS (concerned with BALANCE) and the COCHLEA (concerned with hearing).

inoculation one type of immunization that involves introducing, usually by injection, a small quantity of a modified harmful substance into the body so that the IMMUNE SYSTEM can build resistance to the unmodified form. VACCINATION is a type of inoculation.

insomnia, or sleeplessness the inability to fall or to remain asleep. There are many possible causes, including worry, an uncomfortable bed or surroundings, or undigested food.

instinct an inborn drive, including such aspects of behavior as sexuality and aggression.

insulin a hormone secreted by the PANCREAS. It is essential to regulation of the amount of sugar in the body. Inappropriate response to or abnormally low secretion of insulin causes DIABETES mellitus which can be treated with insulin injections.

intelligence quotient (IQ) an index of "intelligence" arrived at by comparing answers to any of several standard tests with those normalized for age.

intensive care the carefully monitored and continuous treatment given to a patient who is critically ill. For such care the patient may be placed in a specialized section of the hospital.

interferon a protein produced by animal cells after they have been infected by a VIRUS. It serves to slow down the multiplication and spread of the virus.

intervertebral disks disk-shaped pieces of tough cartilage located between the vertebral bones that make up the spinal column.

intestines the alimentary tract from the stomach to the anus, also called the gut, consisting of the DUODENUM, JEJUNUM, ILEUM, CECUM, COLON and RECTUM.

intramuscular within a muscle.

intrauterine device (IUD) a small metallically or hormonally impregnated piece of looped plastic placed within the womb to prevent IMPLANTATION of a fertilized ovum. It is used as a method of

CONTRACEPTION.

intravenous refers to a process whereby a needle or a CATHETER is introduced into a vein.

intravenous pyelogram (IVP) an X-ray picture of the KIDNEYS, made visible after injection of a radiopaque dye.

introvert the psychological term for a person who is more concerned with his or her own thoughts than with external events. The opposite type is called an EXTROVERT.

in-vitro fertilization the technique used to fertilize an OVUM outside a woman's reproductive tract, as the first step toward producing what is popularly known as a TEST-TUBE BABY.

iodine a nonmetallic element which, in small quantities, is essential to health. It is needed by the THYROID GLAND to produce the hormone thyroxine. Lack of iodine in adults leads to GOITER and HYPOTHYROIDISM. In babies its absence may lead to physical defects and mental retardation (CRETINISM). A weak solution of iodine in alcohol is used as an antiseptic for cuts and abrasions.

ion an electrically charged atom or molecule.

ionizing radiation radiation that is sufficiently powerful to break up substances into IONS.

IQ *see* INTELLIGENCE QUOTIENT.

iris the ring of tissue in front of the lens of the EYE which contracts or relaxes its aperture to control the amount of light that enters the eye.

iron a metallic chemical element essential to human life. It is present in hemoglobin, myoglobin and in certain enzymes. Lack of iron leads to anemia.

irradiation the process of submitting a tissue or substance to radiation in the form of heat, radioactive particles or X rays.

ischemia reduced blood supply to a part of the body. As a result, there is also a shortfall of oxygen and nutrients to that part, which may lead to the death of the tissues involved. It is usually caused by diseased blood vessels, and commonly develops in ARTERIOSCLEROSIS.

islets of Langerhans

islets of Langerhans groups of endocrine cells in the PANCREAS, some of which (the beta-cells) produce INSULIN.

isotope a form of an element which has two or more atomic forms with different masses (because of different numbers of neutrons). Radioactive isotopes, or RADIOISOTOPES, are sometimes used in the diagnosis or treatment of diseases.

IUD *see* INTRAUTERINE DEVICE.

J

Jacksonian epilepsy a particular type of EPILEPSY in which convulsions are characterized by originating in the fingers, toes or lips, and then "march" (spread) to adjacent muscles.

Jacob, François a French geneticist who worked with Jacques MONOD to formulate the basis of the theory of the GENETIC CODE.

Jarvik, Robert Koffler (1946–) an American physician who is famed for the invention and successful application of an artificial heart. It was in 1982 that his "Jarvik-7" was introduced into the body of a retired dentist named Barney Clark, who lived on for a further 112 days, succumbing to multiple organ failure, although his new heart was beating as strongly as ever. A later patient lived for 12 months after the implantation of a "Jarvik-7" in 1984.

jaundice a symptom characterized by yellowish skin, blood and tissues. It results from an excess of bilirubin (a yellow bile pigment) in the blood, and is a symptom of liver disease (usually HEPATITIS), hemolytic disease, or obstruction of the biliary system.

jaw comprises two bones, the maxilla (upper jaw) and the movable mandible (lower jaw).

jejunum part of the small intestine that joins the DUODENUM to the ILEUM. About four feet long, it is the site of both DIGESTION and absorption. After the food has been sufficiently broken down, it is transported to the liver by the lymphatic vessels and hepatic portal vein.

Jenner, Edward (1749–1823) an English physician who developed VACCINATION and vanquished SMALLPOX. Jenner found that the milder disease of cowpox seemed to protect people from smallpox. Accordingly, he infected an eight-year-old boy with cowpox matter and six weeks later inoculated him with smallpox virus. The boy remained healthy.

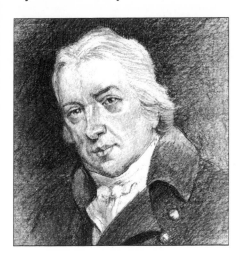

jet lag the disorientation and disruption of the normal CIRCADIAN RHYTHM that a person experiences when flying through several time zones in high-speed aircraft. As a result, the traveler may want to sleep during the day and be lively at night. It may take some days for the rhythm to adapt.

joint the point of ARTICULATION between two bones, such as the hip joint or the elbow. The term is also used for the immovable junction between two or more bones, as in the fused joints between the bones of the skull.

jugular vein any one of four veins that carry blood from the head and neck back to the heart.

Jung, Carl Gustav (1875–1961) a Swiss psychiatrist and psychologist who was the founder of analytical psychology. For many years closely associated with SIGMUND FREUD, he shared with him the conviction that the conscious and unconscious mind had a paramount effect on human behavior. But later, Jung came to the conclusion that Freud placed too much emphasis on sexual instincts in the origins of neuroses. Jung proposed the theory that a deep level of unconsciousness, which he called the collective unconscious, was the primal guiding force of all humanity.

K

keloid   the thickened replacement skin, a type of SCAR tissue, that is sometimes produced to a greater degree than is necessary for healing at the site of a wound.

Kepler, Johannes (1571–1630)   a German astronomer who evolved three laws of planetary motion, and was noted for his research into optics. His knowledge of the anatomy of the eye, combined with his studies into the geometry of rays, enabled him to show that an image of the perceived object was formed on the retina, and not on the lens, as was previously believed.

keratin   a fibrous protein that makes up some hard tissues of the body, such as nails on the fingers and toes. It also occurs as the chief component of hair and in the outer layer of the skin.

ketosis   a condition that occurs during starvation or during a diabetic crisis, when fat instead of sugar is used up for providing energy. This results in abnormal amounts of ketones (substances formed when fatty acids are broken down) being produced. The result may be a slight smell of acetone on the breath.

kidney   one of two organs located in the upper, rear abdomen which filter blood and excrete waste products and excess fluid as urine.

kidney stone   a renal CALCULUS.

kiss of life   a colloquial term for mouth-to-mouth resuscitation which is administered after a person has stopped breathing. Air is gently breathed into a patient's mouth and lungs — once it has been established that the airway is not blocked — in a regular manner so that oxygenation of the blood continues until the patient's lungs begin working again.

knee   the joint in the leg between the thighbone (FEMUR) and the two bones of the lower leg, the TIBIA and FIBULA.

knee jerk   the REFLEX "jump" of the lower leg that is the result of the knee's being tapped with a small hammer just below the kneecap.

knock-knee (medical name, genu valgum)   a deformity of the leg bones in which the knees of a standing person touch although the ankles remain apart — the lower legs are curved outward. It may result from the bone disease RICKETS.

Koch, Robert (1843–1910) an outstanding German bacteriologist who spent a lifetime endeavoring to control TUBERCULOSIS. He first proved that tuberculosis is chronically infectious, and in 1882 announced his positive identification of the bacillus that causes the disease. In 1905 he was awarded the Nobel Prize in physiology and medicine for this achievement.

Kühne, Wilhelm (1837–1900) a German physiologist who spent many years trying to unlock the secrets of vision. He developed a process which he named optography, using the eye of a rabbit as a camera and its retina as his photographic film. By this means he managed to capture and retain on the dried retina an image of the rabbit's last perceived object.

kyphosis a condition in which the spine is abnormally curved. The resulting deformity is commonly called HUNCHBACK.

L

Laban, Rudolf (1879–1958) a German dancer, choreographer, and teacher of modern dance. He devised a system, which he called Labanotation, for recording simultaneous physical movements, which found application in anatomical studies. In this system, by varying the length, shape, and shading of rectangles, he could indicate a movement's speed, direction, and height from the floor.

labor the process of CHILDBIRTH by which the FETUS and PLACENTA (afterbirth) are delivered from the womb. The first stage of labor refers to the preliminary contractions of the womb; the second stage is completed with the delivery of the baby; the third stage of labor involves the expulsion of the placenta.

labyrinth another name for the convoluted channels and tissues that together make up the INNER EAR.

lacrimal gland the tear gland located in the upper, outer corner of each eye socket. It secretes a salty fluid (tears) that keeps the eyeball moist, clean and free from dust particles. Tears are also mildly bactericidal, and so combat potentially harmful germs.

lacrimation production of tears by the LACRIMAL GLAND, in response to irritation of the eyeball or as an emotional reaction.

lactation production of milk from the mammary glands (BREASTS) of a mother to feed her baby. It occurs in response to the presence of the pituitary hormone PROLACTIN, of which the production is stimulated by the baby's sucking.

lactic acid a colorless liquid formed in milk by the bacterial fermentation of sugars. It is also produced in the human body in the muscles during strenuous exercise, after the body has used up the available oxygen to convert carbohydrates, such as glucose, into energy. An accumulation of lactic acid in the muscles causes the spasms of cramp.

Lamarck, Jean-Baptiste de (1744−1829) a French naturalist who became a pioneer of modern biology. In his *Zoological Philosophy* (1809) he advanced the theory that species are constantly changing through individual evolution passed on to the next generation as basis for further evolution. His seven-volume *Natural History of Invertebrates* (1815−1822) became the basis of modern invertebrate zoology.

lameness (medical name, claudication) may be the result of a hereditary handicap, injury, or of poor circulation in the legs. Occasional limping, termed intermittent claudication, with pain in the legs, may result from arterial disease.

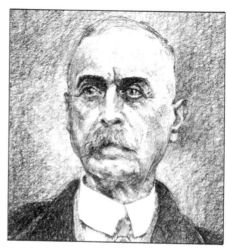

Landsteiner, Karl (1868−1943) an Austrian-born American pathologist who discovered various human BLOOD GROUPS. He discovered groups A, B, AB, and O, and later identified, with A. S. Wiener, the RH

(RHESUS) FACTOR. He also showed that some blood groups are incompatible with others. In 1930 he was awarded the Nobel Prize in physiology and medicine.

Langer's lines a term used to describe the visible alignment of the subcutaneous connective tissue (of the skin). The lines are clearly evident as the creases in the palm of the hand. Surgeons prefer to make operation incisions parallel to such lines because any subsequent scarring is thereby minimized.

lanolin a fatty substance obtained from the wool of sheep. Because it is easily absorbed by the skin, it is used in ointments to soothe skin disorders.

lanugo the layer of fine downy hair that covers a fetus; some lanugo may persist for a few days after birth.

laparoscopy examination of the interior of the abdomen with a lighted optical tube called a laparoscope. The patient is anesthetized, a small incision is made in the abdomen, and the tube inserted. The technique is used particularly to examine the ovaries and Fallopian tubes.

laparotomy a surgical operation to open the abdominal cavity. It may be performed to examine the organs in the cavity (termed an exploratory laparotomy) or as a prelude to further abdominal surgery.

laryngectomy a surgical operation to remove all or part of the LARYNX (voice box), usually because of the presence of a cancerous tumor. A permanent opening is left in the TRACHEA (windpipe) through which the patient can breathe. Speech can sometimes be restored with training and practice.

laryngitis inflammation of the LARYNX, caused either by bacteria or a virus. The vocal cords are affected and the voice becomes husky or disappears altogether.

larynx the structure within the trachea in which the basic sounds of speech are produced.

laxatives DRUGS that stimulate the emptying of the bowels. They may be used as treatment for constipation.

lead a HEAVY METAL, compounds of which are poisonous. Lead poisoning is cumulative in effect, and is remarkably common, particularly in children (who tend to lick objects painted with lead paint).

learning disabilities in children are many and varied. They include difficulty in reading, writing, and mathematics, as well as poor concentration, memory and physical coordination, allied sometimes to constant misbehavior. Causes may lie in brain damage, or damage to the nervous system, mental handicap, unsuspected deafness, or merely a lack of experience and opportunity to learn. Treatment depends on diagnosis.

lecithin any one of a group of chemicals made up of fatty acids, phosphoric acid and a nitrogen base. It is found in many animal tissues, especially egg yolk, and is a constituent of nerve cells and brain tissue.

leech a bloodsucking parasitic worm that was once used in medicine as a means of bloodletting.

Leeuwenhoek, Anton van (1632–1723) a Dutch amateur scientist who, with home-made MICROSCOPES, was able to discover and describe in detail microorganisms and red blood cells. In 1677 he reported the existence of spermatozoa, and eleven years later demonstrated that red blood cells change shape to squeeze through small arteries.

left-handedness a tendency to prefer to use the left hand when most people would use only the right. About ten per cent of people are left-handed, and many of them are also left-footed.

legionnaire's disease a contagious bacterial disease of the lungs. It was named for an American Legion conference in Pennsylvania in 1976, when 29 out of 182 people who attended the conference hotel and were affected, died. The symptoms are those of an acute form of PNEUMONIA. It is caused by a bacterium that lives in moist places, especially water systems or humidified ventilation systems.

lens a transparent doubly-curved disk in the EYE which focuses light on to the retina. If it functions imperfectly, a supplementary lens can be provided in the form of EYE-GLASSES to correct and improve vision.

leprosy a progressive bacterial disease of the skin, peripheral nerves and nasal tissue. Once known as Hansen's disease, it is probably spread by droplets from the nose and mouth of an infected person, but although it is infectious in and to children, it is far less so in and to adults.

lesbianism   female HOMOSEXUALITY.

lesion   any internal or external abnormality in a tissue. It includes wounds, sores, blisters and tumors.

lethargy   an abnormal feeling of fatigue and listlessness. It may occur during convalescence or be a symptom of a disorder.

leukemia   a type of CANCER marked by the presence of an abnormally large number of white blood cells which seem much less than usually capable of defending against infection.

leukocyte   the medical name for a white BLOOD CELL.

libido   a psychological term for an individual's urge for sexual fulfillment.

life expectancy   figures differ from country to country, but in the United States the current average life expectancy at birth for both sexes is more than 70 years. Such statistics are used in many ways around the world, particularly to define areas whose populations are especially liable to early death.

life-support machine   any specialized machine designed to sustain a human life artificially when, without such support, death would rapidly follow; for instance, following a serious disease or injury.

ligament   CONNECTIVE TISSUE that binds bones together and holds other body tissues in place. Ligaments usually take the form of bands or sheets. Some have muscles attached to them, in which case they may function in a similar manner to tendons.

ligature   a thread, wire or cord used to tie round a vessel or constrict a tube in the body.

limbic system   that part of the brain that links the CORTEX (the outer layer) with the HYPOTHALAMUS in the center of the brain. It is associated with basic emotions such as hunger and sexual pleasure.

Lind, James (1716–1794)   a Scottish physician who became the founder of nautical medicine. He recommended that fresh fruit and especially lime or lemon juice should be part of every sailor's daily

lipid

diet and, as a result, SCURVY (caused by a deficiency in VITAMIN C) was virtually eradicated from the British fleet. Lind was also concerned with other aspects of naval health, including ventilation, overcrowding, and bad water supplies.

lipid   any one of a group of FATS and fatlike substances in foods and in the body. They are an important source of reserve energy.

lipoprotein   any one of a group of simple proteins to which a LIPID molecule is attached.

lips   generally, the two fleshy folds that surround the mouth.

Lister, Joseph   (1827–1912) English surgeon who pioneered the idea of antiseptic surgery. Initially he used a solution of carbolic acid (phenol) for cleaning wounds, and by 1867 had introduced a spray of carbolic acid to kill germs in the operating theater. He later combined this with the German Robert Koch's technique of sterilizing surgical instruments and dressings.

litholapaxy   one method of removing a stone, or CALCULUS, from the urinary bladder without making a surgical incision. After examining the inside of the bladder with a cystoscope, the surgeon crushes the stone by LITHOTRITY. The fragments are flushed away.

lithotomy   a surgical operation to remove a large stone, or CALCULUS, from the urinary bladder or elsewhere. Smaller stones may be removed by LITHOLAPAXY.

lithotrity   the crushing of a stone, or CALCULUS, in the urinary bladder or elsewhere effected with an instrument called a lithotrite.

liver   the principal site of METABOLISM in the body, and physically the largest glandular organ. It is located immediately beneath the DIAPHRAGM. Blood carrying the usable products of digestion flows directly to the liver, where glucose is converted by GLYCOGEN for storage, used to form amino acids, or metabolized to FATTY ACIDS. The liver is a major site for lipid (fat) metabolism. Some amino acids are broken down; others are converted to proteins. Toxins are also neutralized. Waste products, including urea, ammonia and carbon dioxide, are removed via the bloodstream for excretion from the kidneys or lungs. The liver

110

also breaks down blood cells and excretes waste products as BILE to the GALL BLADDER.

lobe a rounded, projecting part of the body, such as an ear lobe. It can also be a subdivision of a bodily organ, such as a lobe of the brain, the lungs or the liver.

lobotomy surgery now performed rarely, to cut through the white matter forming the frontal lobe of the brain.

lochia the vaginal discharge of tissue, mucus, and blood that continues for three or four weeks after CHILDBIRTH.

lockjaw an archaic name for TETANUS.

locomotion movement by voluntary means, principally walking or running.

locomotor ataxia a symptom of tabes dorsalis, a form of advanced SYPHILIS that attacks the spinal cord and nerve fibers. It represents a lack of coordination in the muscles of the body, particularly in the legs.

Loewi, Otto (1873–1961) an Austrian physiologist who proved that separate nerve cells communicate with each other mainly by chemical rather than electrical means, as had up to that time been supposed.

longsightedness *see* HYPEROPIA.

loop of Henle a thin tubule of each nephron in the KIDNEY that bends sharply back on itself in the shape of a hairpin.

louse a wingless insect, three species of which are parasitic on human beings. One lives on the body and in the hair; one, the head louse, lives on the scalp; and the third, the CRAB LOUSE, lives in the pubic hair. Lice cause itching of the skin and possible infection through scratching the irritation.

lumbago a general term for pain in the lower back. There are many possible causes, including disorders of the spine or in other parts of the body, including gynecological disorders and kidney problems. Among other likely causes are FIBROSITIS and SLIPPED DISK. Lumbago is also a general word for BACKACHE.

lumbar puncture a diagnostic technique in which a hollow needle is inserted at the base of the spine to remove CEREBROSPINAL FLUID from the spinal canal.

LUNGS

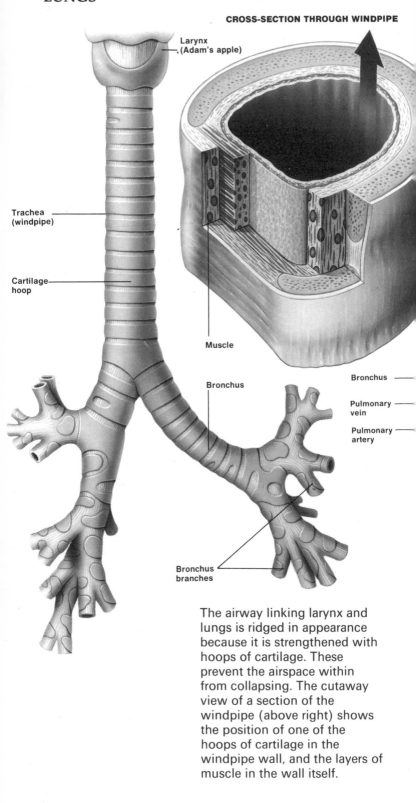

CROSS-SECTION THROUGH WINDPIPE

Larynx (Adam's apple)

Trachea (windpipe)

Cartilage hoop

Muscle

Bronchus

Bronchus

Pulmonary vein

Pulmonary artery

Bronchus branches

The airway linking larynx and lungs is ridged in appearance because it is strengthened with hoops of cartilage. These prevent the airspace within from collapsing. The cutaway view of a section of the windpipe (above right) shows the position of one of the hoops of cartilage in the windpipe wall, and the layers of muscle in the wall itself.

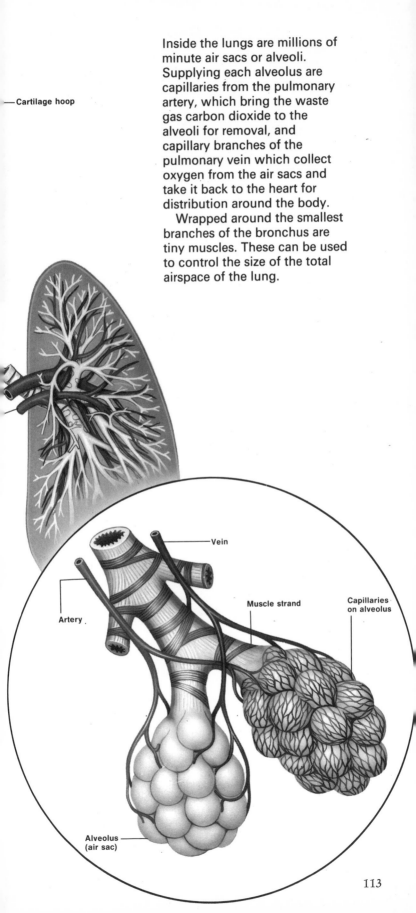

Cartilage hoop

Inside the lungs are millions of minute air sacs or alveoli. Supplying each alveolus are capillaries from the pulmonary artery, which bring the waste gas carbon dioxide to the alveoli for removal, and capillary branches of the pulmonary vein which collect oxygen from the air sacs and take it back to the heart for distribution around the body.

Wrapped around the smallest branches of the bronchus are tiny muscles. These can be used to control the size of the total airspace of the lung.

Vein

Muscle strand

Capillaries on alveolus

Artery

Alveolus (air sac)

113

lumen   the inner open space of a blood vessel, intestine or other tube, or of the doughnut-shaped prostate gland in men.

lung   one of two large, lobed organs in the chest. Air is drawn into the lungs through the trachea during breathing, and it is in them that blood takes up oxygen and releases carbon dioxide.

lung cancer   a disorder resulting from the presence of malignant cells in the lung, generally as a TUMOR. It can produce secondary cancers (by METASTASIS) in other parts of the body. Initial symptoms are a cough from which there may be blood-stained sputum. Pneumonia or the collapse of a lung may follow.

lupus   any one of a number of chronic diseases that affect the skin. Lupus vulgaris is tuberculosis of the skin, marked by facial lesions. Lupus erythematosus is an inflammatory disease that attacks the connective tissue. It is characterized by a scaly red rash on the face.

luteinizing hormone   a HORMONE secreted by the pituitary gland. In women, it stimulates ovulation and helps to form the CORPUS LUTEUM from a ruptured ovarian follicle. In men, it helps the development of the TESTES.

lymph   a colorless body fluid that has its own circulatory system; involved mainly in the metabolism of fats, lymph also helps remove bacteria and other particles from the body.

lymphatic system   comprises a network throughout the body of vessels that carry LYMPH from between cells in the tissues to the bloodstream. Glands that produce lymph are located at intervals along the lymph vessels, particularly in the armpits and groin.

lymphocyte   a type of white BLOOD CELL.

M

MacLeod, John James Rickard (1876 – 1935)   a British physiologist who helped Frederick BANTING in his discovery of INSULIN for use in the treatment of DIABETES. At the time of the discovery (1922) Professor MacLeod was head of the Physiology Department at the University of Toronto. The two men shared the 1923

Nobel Prize in physiology and medicine for their efforts.

macrophage any large cell of the type that engulfs other cells (PHAGOCYTE) which is present in the blood, bone marrow, connective tissue and LYMPHATIC SYSTEM.

Magendie, François (1783–1855) a French physiologist who was a pioneer in experimental physiology in France. In 1822 he was able to prove the correctness of Scottish physician Charles Bell's earlier theories regarding the functions of the motor and sensory nerves, and thereafter claimed the original discovery as his own.

malabsorption syndrome a group of symptoms produced in a patient whose body is unable to absorb essential nutrients from food. These symptoms include weight loss, anemia, diarrhea and vitamin deficiency diseases. There are many possible causes, including enzyme deficiency, damage to the stomach and intestines, CYSTIC FIBROSIS and CELIAC DISEASE.

malaise a general feeling of listlessness and lethargy without evidence of any specific illness. It may indicate the onset of infection.

malaria, or ague an infectious disease, common in the tropics, of which the symptoms are chill, sweating and fever. It is caused by a parasite called *Plasmodium* and transmitted by the bites of the *Anopheles* mosquito.

malformation a defective formation, especially a deformation present at birth, classified as a CONGENITAL DISORDER.

malignant a process of disease is so described if it is severe, progressive and resistant to treatment. In reference to CANCER, it implies the capacity for METASTASIS.

malleus the largest and outermost of three small bones in the middle ear, the others being the incus and the stapes.

malnutrition a lack of adequate nutrition. This may arise from shortage of food, an ill-balanced diet, or defects in the digestive system.

Malpighi, Marcello (1628–1694) an Italian anatomist who became known as the father of histology, the founder of modern anatomy and botany, and a pioneer of microscopic research. Among his achievements was the discovery of capillaries on the surface of the lungs, and research into the structure of skin tissue.

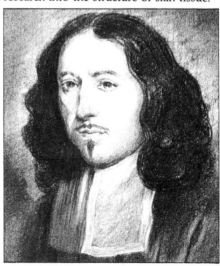

mammography examination of a woman's breast by X rays in order to detect any abnormal growths.

mammoplasty the alteration of the size or shape of a woman's breast by PLASTIC SURGERY.

mandible the lower bone of the JAW.

mania a disorder of mood characterized by expansiveness, excitability and possibly decreased sleep. It can be symptomatic of MANIC-DEPRESSIVE ILLNESS or of one of several drugs.

manic-depressive illness a mental disorder characterized either by episodes of MANIA or by episodes of mania alternating with periods of DEPRESSION. It can be treated with drugs.

marrow the jelly-like substance occupying the spaces in bones, also called bone marrow, where blood cells are produced.

masochism the derivation of pleasure from pain inflicted either by oneself or by others. In sexual masochism, pain is required for sexual gratification.

masseter the cheek muscle which closes the jaws and facilitates chewing.

mastectomy the removal of part or all of a woman's BREAST by surgery, usually to arrest the development of CANCER.

mastication, or chewing the breaking down of food into small particles in the mouth. There it is mixed with SALIVA, which starts the digestive process.

mastitis inflammation of a woman's breast. The cause may be infection or a hormone imbalance. Chronic cystic mastitis is a common condition characterized by benign cysts or lumps. Puerperal mastitis is an acute bacterial infection that may occur in nursing mothers.

mastoid a projecting, spongy air-filled bone behind the ear. The air cells inside it are linked to the MIDDLE EAR.

masturbation manipulation of the genital organs, usually one's own, in order to achieve ORGASM without sexual intercourse.

maxilla the upper JAWbone.

measles (medical name, rubeola) a contagious virus disease that commonly affects children. Symptoms start with high fever, a sore throat and a running nose. This is followed by small white spots in the mouth and a pinkish-orange rash that soon covers the whole body. An effective VACCINE is available.

meconium the dark greenish, thick pasty FECES passed by a baby during the first few days of life.

Medawar, Peter B. (1915 –) a Brazilian-born British biologist who, with his colleague and mentor Frank Burnet, was jointly awarded the 1960 Nobel Prize in physiology and medicine for research into immunological tolerance.

medulla the innermost core of an organ or structure.

medulla oblongata, sometimes called simply the medulla the swelling of the spinal cord that forms the lowest part of the brainstem.

meiosis the process of cell division — universal in plants and animals — by which a human cell containing forty-six chromosomes divides to produce two sperm cells or two egg cells with twenty-three chromosomes each.

melanin the natural dark pigment that occurs in the hair, skin and iris of the eye.

melanoma a black or brown MALIGNANT tumor that starts from a cell which normally produces MELANIN. Any dark swelling, mole or other skin blemish that appears to be increasing in size should be shown to a physician. Treatment may be by surgery or CHEMOTHERAPY, or both.

melasma   a condition in which brown patches appear on the forehead and cheeks, made worse by sunlight. It appears in some women who are pregnant or who take contraceptive pills.

membrane   any thin, usually flexible, layer of tissue which lines, covers, or partitions internal parts of the body. Membranes can be as thin as two molecules (as in a phospholipid membrane) or as tough as the protective dura membrane that covers the spinal cord.

memory   the ability of the brain to store and recall sensations and knowledge from past experience. Distant, recent, or immediate recall is controlled by different parts of the brain. Loss of memory is called AMNESIA.

menarche   the first episode of menstruation in a pubescent girl.

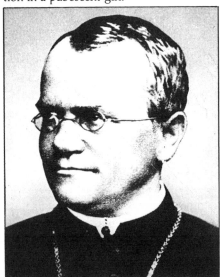

Mendel, Gregor Johann (1822–1884) an Austrian monk and botanist who discovered what was later called Mendel's law of HEREDITY, by crossbreeding different strains of plants, mostly peas. He discovered that the offspring of certain strains would display "dominant" and "recessive" traits in fixed ratios.

Ménière's disease   a disorder of the inner ear characterized by recurrent episodes of VERTIGO, TINNITUS and deafness. Onset can be at any age, but is most common in the fifties. Causes of the disorder are poorly understood.

meninges the three membranes that cover and protect the central nervous system — the brain and the spinal cord. They are the dura (outer), arachnoid (middle) and pia (inner) membranes.

meningitis inflammation of the MENINGES. There are a number of possible causes, including bacterial, viral and fungal infections. Symptoms include a high fever, vomiting and severe headache.

meningocele the protrusion of the MENINGES through an opening in the skull or backbone. The condition is congenital.

menopause the termination of MENSTRUATION and thus of the reproductive phase of life in women. It usually occurs between the ages of forty-five and fifty-five. It is accompanied by some other physical and psychological effects.

menorrhagia abnormally heavy bleeding during MENSTRUATION; periods may also last longer. The many possible causes include high blood pressure or a growth in the ovary.

menstrual cycle the regular monthly sequence of hormonal changes that affect a woman after puberty and result in MENSTRUATION. The cycle starts as the lining of the WOMB (endometrium) thickens and a follicle in the ovary matures. The OVUM is released about halfway through the cycle (ovulation). If it is fertilized, it implants in the endometrium and PREGNANCY begins. If not, menstruation occurs as the endometrial tissue is shed.

menstruation the monthly discharge of blood and the lining of the WOMB through the vagina in women of childbearing age. Each menstrual period lasts between three and seven days. Menstruation continues from MENARCHE to MENOPAUSE, usually ceasing only during PREGNANCY.

mental disorder any disorder in behavior or function of mental origin, whether caused by psychological, chemical or biological factors.

mental retardation, or mental deficiency subnormal intelligence. It may be present at birth, or it may be caused by brain injury or disease.

mercury a poisonous HEAVY METAL used in many clinical thermometers.

mesentery is a fold of the PERITONEUM

extending from the posterior abdominal wall that encircles most of the intestines, and connects the intestine to the abdominal wall.

mesomorph a standardized type of body shape differentiated from ECTOMORPH and ENDOMORPH. A mesomorph, typically, has a strong skeletal frame, which may be well muscled, and is neither tall and thin nor fat.

metabolism the combination of physical and chemical processes that occur in the body at the molecular level in order to maintain life.

metacarpal one of the five bones of the palm of the HAND.

metastasis the spread of a disease or disease-causing agent from one part of the body to another via the bloodstream or the lymphatic system. The term is most commonly used to describe the internal spread of CANCER.

metatarsal one of the five long bones in the foot. Metatarsals form the framework of the flexible arch linking the heel bones to the toes.

microbe a living, microscopic organism, especially one that causes disease.

microorganism any living animal or plant of microscopic size, such as a BACTERIUM or a PROTOZOAN.

microscope an optical instrument that produces a magnified image of a small object. In an ordinary mechanical microscope the object to be studied is placed on a glass slide and viewed by means of two or more lenses. It is used extensively in medicine.

microvilli the microscopic fingerlike projections extending from the surface of many internal CELL membranes.

micturition a medical term for urination, or the passing of URINE.

midbrain (medical name, mesencephalon) a stalk of nerve fibers that is the main connection between the CEREBRUM of the brain and the hindbrain.

middle ear part of the EAR that contains the EARDRUM and the three ossicles (sound-conducting bones), which connect with the INNER EAR. It is linked to the back of the throat by the EUSTACHIAN TUBE.

migraine an extremely severe, recurrent type of HEADACHE, usually on one side of the head only, and associated with nausea, vomiting, light sensitivity and visual disturbances. It is thought to be triggered off, in many sufferers, by certain kinds of food, drink, or even specific events. It may be caused by a vascular abnormality.

milk the liquid produced from a mother's BREAST to feed her newborn baby. True milk begins to flow a few days after the birth. Before that, a milky fluid called COLOSTRUM is secreted by the breasts.

milk teeth a child's first set of twenty teeth.

miscarriage the unexpected loss of a FETUS from the WOMB before the seventh month of pregnancy. It is also called a spontaneous ABORTION.

mite a minute animal PARASITE related to spiders and scorpions. It can live on the skin or in the hair, and may carry disease.

mitochondria tiny bodies located in the cytoplasm of a cell metabolism.

mitosis a process of cell division in which the nucleus divides to produce two "daughter" cells, each having the same number of CHROMOSOMES as the parent cells.

molars the large chewing TEETH situated at the back of the jaw.

mole a dark spot or area of pigmentation in the skin. Moles are almost always harmless. A potentially dangerous complication is the development of a MELANOMA.

mongolism *see* DOWN'S SYNDROME.

moniliasis another name for the fungal infection CANDIDIASIS.

monocyte a LEUKOCYTE with a large nucleus and more cytoplasm than most other white BLOOD CELLS.

Monod, Jacques Lucien (1910–1976) and **Jacob, François** (1920–) two French scientists who worked together at the Pasteur Institute to jointly formulate a theory (since proved substantially correct) that metabolism, growth, and development within cells is controlled by genes. Monod was essentially a biochemist and Jacob a geneticist.

mononucleosis, or infectious mononucleosis alternative names for GLANDULAR FEVER.

Montessori, Maria (1870–1952)   an Italian physician and educationalist who developed the world-famous method of bringing up children known as the Montessori Method. She believed that a child should be allowed to develop naturally by encouraging his or her initiative and natural abilities through individual guidance rather than strict control.

Morgan, Thomas Hunt (1866–1945) an American biologist who, in experiments with the fruit fly *Drosophila*, showed that CHROMOSOMES were responsible for hereditary effects, that combinations of GENES were responsible for individual characteristics, and that such combinations could be traced to specific groups of genes which it would eventually be possible to map. His importance to modern genetics would be difficult to exaggerate.

morning sickness   a condition to which some women are prone during the early months of PREGNANCY, involving nausea (mostly on getting up in the morning).

morphine   an extremely powerful ANALGESIC and SEDATIVE. Like other drugs derived from opium, it is also addictive.

Morton, William Thomas Green (1819–1868)   an American dentist who first successfully demonstrated to the scientific world the use of ether as an ANESTHETIC for surgical operations. The demonstration took place in 1846 on a young man in need of surgery. Morton's attempts to obtain the credit for discovering anesthesia failed because he was sued by his rivals.

morula   a round mass of embryonic cells resulting from the division and development of a just-fertilized egg.

mosquito   a flying, bloodsucking insect equipped with a long, sharp proboscis (or beak), which is specially adapted to pierce the skin. Some are carriers of dangerous diseases such as MALARIA, YELLOW FEVER, and ENCEPHALITIS.

motion sickness   *see* TRAVEL SICKNESS.

motor cortex   a section of the thin layer of gray matter (CORTEX) that comprises the two hemispheres of the brain. It controls voluntary muscles in various parts of the body.

motor end-plate   the flattened end of a motor nerve fiber at the point where it comes into contact with a MUSCLE fiber.

motor neurone disease   a group of allied disorders of the nervous system. It involves progressive atrophy of the motor nerves, resulting in the wasting of the muscles they supply.

mountain sickness   *see* ALTITUDE SICKNESS.

mouth-to-mouth resuscitation, or the kiss of life   a form of ARTIFICIAL RESPIRATION.

mouth ulcer   a small ULCER in the MUCOUS MEMBRANE of the mouth or tongue.

MS   *see* MULTIPLE SCLEROSIS.

mucous colitis   inflammation of the MUCOUS MEMBRANES lining the COLON.

mucous membrane   a membrane containing glands that secrete MUCUS. Such membranes line body passages and organs that are open to external infection, such as the nose, mouth, intestines and vagina.

mucus   a slimy secretion produced by MUCUS MEMBRANES. It lubricates body linings, keeps them moist, and protects against infection.

Muller, Hermann Joseph (1890–1967) an American geneticist who was awarded the 1946 Nobel Prize in physiology and medicine for his pioneering work on the artificial mutation of genes through radiation with X rays.

multiple sclerosis, or disseminated sclerosis   a disorder that attacks parts of the brain and the spinal cord. Many small, white, hard patches appear scattered throughout the area and interfere with the nerve pathways. Outward symptoms include visual problems, tremor, bladder dysfunction, weakness of the limbs, and other neurological problems. The disease is chronic and progressive, yet it is characterized by long periods of remission and recurrences. The cause is unknown, although there is a familial predisposition. On average, a patient lives on for twenty years after diagnosis, eventually succumbing to an infection.

mumps (medical name, parotitis)   a contagious virus disease that mainly attacks the salivary glands, and sometimes involves the MENINGES and pancreas. It more commonly affects children and teenagers, and is marked by swelling and pain in the glands and organs involved. In males the testicles are sometimes affected.

murmur an abnormal noise from the heart, which may indicate VALVULAR DISEASE OF THE HEART.

muscle the tissue that effects movement in the body. There are three types of muscle tissue: skeletal muscle (also called striated or striped), which is under voluntary control; smooth muscle, which is not controlled consciously; and cardiac muscle, which occurs only in the heart.

muscle relaxants DRUGS commonly used to prepare the body for surgery; they may also constitute therapy for some kinds of muscular spasm.

muscular dystrophy a group of disorders which have in common the slow but progressive wasting away of the muscles. Massage and physiotherapy are helpful in slowing the wasting process.

mutation is any permanent change in the genetic material of a cell.

mute a person who cannot speak. Mutism may result from disease or an accident to the VOCAL CORDS, or it may follow a STROKE.

myasthenia gravis chronic AUTOIMMUNE DISEASE that affects neural transmission and thus interferes with the nerve impulses that control the muscles, which atrophy. It can be serious if it affects the muscles involved in breathing, but drugs, surgery or sometimes just bed rest can be curative.

myelin the cream-colored fatty substance around the AXON of a nerve fiber.

myelocele the most serious form of SPINA BIFIDA. It is a condition in which the spinal cord protrudes through a hole in the SPINE.

myelogram an X-ray of the spinal canal used in diagnosis.

myocardial infarction a type of HEART ATTACK caused by death of heart muscle tissue after the local blood supply has been interrupted by CORONARY ARTERY DISEASE, spasm or EMBOLISM.

myofibril   a minute fiber that contributes to the muscle fibers.

myopathy   any of a group of diseases in which there is wastage and degeneration of the muscles, but which is not attributed to any defect in the nervous system.

myopia, or shortsightedness   a defect of vision which allows a person to see things in focus only when they are close. Light rays tend to focus in front of the retina, rather than on it, because the eyeball is too long or the lens is too curved.

myxedema   a form of HYPOTHYROIDISM.

myxovirus   a type of VIRUS which includes those that cause INFLUENZA and MUMPS.

N

nail   hard, dead tissue that covers part of the upper surfaces of the fingers and toes. It contains the protein KERATIN.

narcotics   DRUGS that cause sleep; the term usually refers to opium derivatives, which are highly ADDICTIVE.

nasal septum   a thin wall of bone and cartilage in the NOSE that separates the two cavities leading to the nostrils.

nasopharynx   the part of the PHARYNX that lies above the soft palate, and that links the nasal cavities and the throat.

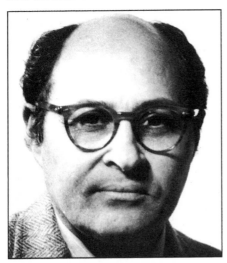

Nathans, Daniel (1928–)   an American microbiologist who showed that genes

naturopathy

could be fully and accurately mapped by managing to divide a carcinogenic virus into eleven identifiable fragments. He shared the 1978 Nobel Prize in physiology and medicine with Hamilton SMITH, who worked independently on genes.

naturopathy   a form of healing that relies on natural means such as sunlight, fresh air and water or massage to achieve a cure. It is classed as an ALTERNATIVE MEDICINE.

nausea   feeling sick, wanting to vomit.

navel   *see* UMBILICUS.

nearsightedness   *see* MYOPIA.

necrosis   the death of an area of tissue. It may occur after an accident, a burn, or disease.

neonate   a newborn child; one generally less than 28 days old.

neoplasm   any abnormal new growth of tissue, BENIGN or MALIGNANT.

nephrolithiasis   the condition of having a CALCULUS in the KIDNEY.

nephrosis   degeneration of kidney tissue, but without inflammation, often causing NEPHROTIC SYNDROME.

nephrotic syndrome   a group of symptoms resulting from damage to the kidney. This causes large quantities of protein to be excreted in the urine. With less protein in the blood, body fluids accumulate in the tissues and cause EDEMA. Swelling and puffiness around the face are accompanied by fatigue, weakness and loss of appetite. Carefully monitored drug treatment may relieve the condition.

nerve   a group of fibers of nervous tissue, concerned with conducting electrochemical impulses.

nerve block   an interruption in the flow of electrical impulses along the nerve fibers. This results in a complete loss of sensation in the affected part, and afterward sometimes a tingling sensation.

nerve cell   *see* NEURON.

nerve fiber   a bundle of long fibers that make up a nerve. There are two types: sensory fibers, which carry messages from various parts of the body to the central nervous system; and motor fibers, which

take command signals from the central nervous system to the glands and muscles.

nervous breakdown   an imprecise non-medical term for a state of mental collapse.

nervous system   the sum total of all neurological tissues in the body. It is normally classified in two parts: the central and peripheral nervous systems. The central nervous system (CNS) consists of the brain and spinal cord. The peripheral nervous systems are sensory-motor or AUTONOMIC; the latter is divided into SYMPATHETIC and PARASYMPATHETIC.

nettlerash, or urticaria   an allergic reaction also called HIVES.

neuralgia   a sharp pain along the course of a nerve or nerves. The cause is often unknown, but it may be due to injury, direct pressure, infection or irritation. Facial neuralgia may be caused by ill-fitting dentures or other dental problems.

neural tube defect   a congenital disorder in which the neural tube forming the brain and spinal cord in the embryo fails to form correctly.

neuritis   inflammation of a nerve, which may or may not be painful.

neuroglia, or glia   the tissue that surrounds, supports and nourishes the NEURONS of the central nervous system.

neuron   a nerve cell, comprising a nerve cell body with branchlike projections called DENDRITES and a stalklike AXON.

neurosis   an emotional or mental disorder sometimes caused by a traumatic event, by internal conflict or by inappropriate ways of dealing with anxiety. It often has physical or behavioral symptoms. Unlike a psychosis a neurosis does not cause a person to lose touch with reality, although neurotic behavior is commonly regarded as "irrational".

neurosurgery   specialized surgery on any part of the nervous system.

neurotransmitters   chemicals released by nerve cells to bridge tiny gaps in the nerve chain called SYNAPSES.

neutrophil   the commonest white blood cell, important in protecting the body against bacterial infections.

NERVES

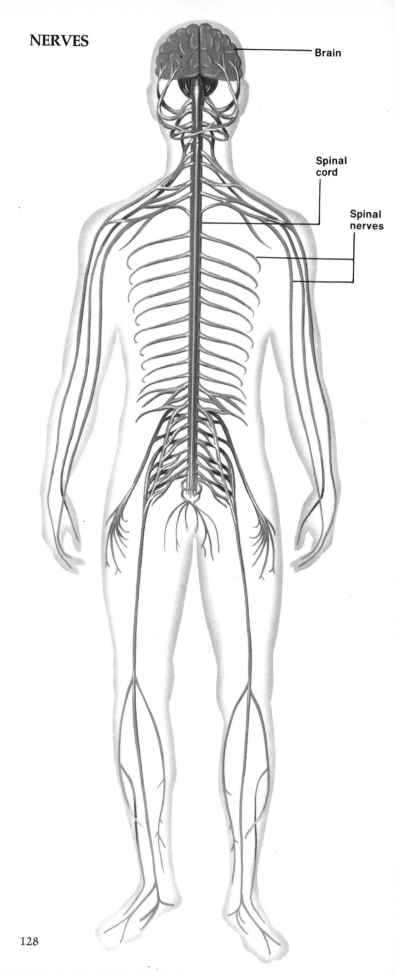

Brain

Spinal cord

Spinal nerves

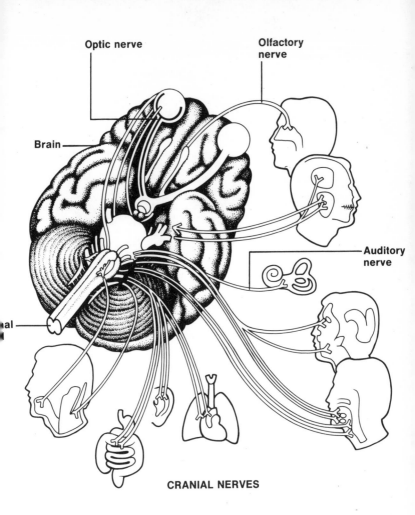

CRANIAL NERVES

Optic nerve

Olfactory nerve

Brain

Auditory nerve

…al

12 pairs of cranial nerves …er the brain from beneath. …ne bring information into the …n from the senses or other …rnal body organs; these are …wn as sensory nerves. …er, motor, nerves send …ormation out to different …ts of the body to initiate action of some kind. The cranial nerves are among the most crucial nerves in the entire nervous system and help control vital activities such as sight, hearing, balance, breathing and digestion.

… nervous system is …mposed of two parts: central … peripheral. The central …vous system is made up of … brain and spinal cord. The …ipheral nervous system …eads out from the spinal …d to all the tissues of the …ly. It includes sensory and …tor nerves, and autonomic …ves which carry impulses to … from involuntary muscles, …ues and glands.

niacin

niacin, or nicotinic acid   a VITAMIN of the B complex which prevents PELLAGRA; it is found particularly in lean meat, milk, liver, yeast, eggs and wheat germ.

nicotine   a stimulant alkaloid drug present in tobacco. Pure nicotine is extremely poisonous, causing vomiting, weakness, collapse and death.

night blindness   lack of, or defective, vision at night or in dim light. It is caused by lack of the protein pigment rhodopsin (visual purple) in the light-sensitive RODS in the retina of the eye.

nipple   a raised area in the center of the AREOLA at the tip of the BREAST. In a woman, it is the outlet for milk ducts from the mammary glands. These secrete MILK from the end of PREGNANCY to feed a baby.

nit   the egg of a LOUSE. Nits stick to the hair of an infested person and appear as small white particles.

nitroglycerin,   in medicine, one of several DRUGS called vasodilators which expand blood vessels; it is used to relieve symptoms of ANGINA PECTORIS.

nitrous oxide   one of many anesthetic DRUGS. Its pleasant smell and sometimes euphoric effect have given it the common name "laughing gas."

NMR   *see*   NUCLEAR MAGNETIC RESONANCE.

nocturia   urination at night, especially if excessive.

node   any distinguishable point in a series, or any junction in a network, such as a lymph gland.

nodes of Ranvier   gaps that occur at regular intervals along the myelin sheath of a nerve fiber, exposing the AXON.

nonspecific urethritis (NSU)   a sexually-transmitted disease characterized by inflammation of the URETHRA. Symptoms in women may be mild or absent; in men urination causes pain and there may be a thick, white discharge. Treatment is usually with antibiotic drugs.

norepinephrine, or noradrenaline   one of the two HORMONES produced by the medulla of the ADRENAL GLAND. As a vasoconstrictor it has similar effects to EPINEPHRINE, the other adrenal medullary hormone.

nose the fleshy, cartilaginous protuberance above the mouth on the face, through which air is inhaled and exhaled. The nose houses the nasal passages where the receptors for the sense of smell are located.

nosebleed or epistaxis occurs for many reasons. Injury to the nose, a heavy cold, high blood pressure, or a blood disorder can all cause a nosebleed.

nostrils the two external openings of the NOSE.

NSU *see* NONSPECIFIC URETHRITIS.

nuclear magnetic resonance scan (NMR), or nuclear scanning an imaging technique that presents a visual picture of internal body tissues through the reaction of atomic nuclei to a magnetic field. Electromagnetic signals are fed back to a computer, which analyzes them and stores them in a retrieval system. Diagnosis of some types of tissue damage is possible using the technique.

nucleotide an organic compound made up of a purine or pyramidine base, a sugar, and phosphoric acid, together the major constituents of nucleic acid and genes.

nucleus an important part of a CELL, which in humans contains twenty-three pairs of chromosomes that dominate its function and replication.

nutrition the regulation of health and growth determined solely by the processes of eating, digestion and the assimilation of food.

nystagmus repetitive directional and parallel twitching of both eyes. A person may be born with this neurological disorder, but more commonly it results from disease.

O

obesity the condition of being considerably overweight in proportion to height and build usually caused by overeating.

obsession a persistent idea, experienced as "foreign" and unreasonable but which the sufferer nonetheless cannot lose. A severe obsession may require psychiatric therapy.

obstetrics the branch of medicine concerned with women during PREGNANCY, LABOR and CHILDBIRTH.

obstructive lung disease a condition in which the flow of air to and from the lungs is impeded. It may be caused by any one of many lung diseases, including BRONCHITIS, EMPHYSEMA and ASTHMA.

occipital pertaining to the back of the skull.

occlusion the state of being closed: a blocked artery may thus be described as occluded. The term occlusion is also used in dentistry, describing the closing together of the jaw.

occupational disorder or industrial disease any one of a multitude of disorders associated with specific jobs or industries. They include lung disorders such as SILICOSIS among miners and sand blasters, and ASBESTOSIS among workers in shipyards or the insulation industry; cataracts of the eyes among glassblowers; and BRUCELLOSIS among farm workers and veterinarians.

occupational therapy a form of treatment for the longer-term physically or mentally ill or handicapped, which generally involves some creative project such as woodwork or pottery, so providing purpose and interest — both valuable aids to rehabilitation.

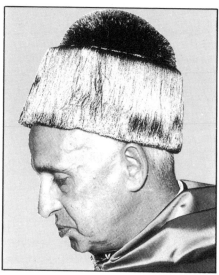

Ochoa, Severo (1905–) a Spanish-born American biochemist who was the first to discover that metabolic energy is stored in or used by the body through high-energy phosphate compounds. For this and his pioneering work with enzymes, he shared the 1956 Nobel Prize in physiology and medicine.

oculist a physician who practices OPHTHALMOLOGY.

Oedipus complex a term used in psychoanalysis to describe a boy's sexual desire for his mother and corresponding jealous feelings toward his father. It is named for the story of Oedipus in Greek mythology. The female equivalent is called an Electra complex.

olecranon the large, pointed end of the ulna (forearm bone) that in some people protrudes at the back of a bent elbow, commonly called the funny bone.

olfactory concerned with the sense of smell. The term is used mostly in connection with the OLFACTORY BULB and the OLFACTORY NERVE.

olfactory bulb the slightly rounded end of the olfactory tract, located in the cranium just above the NOSE. It is connected with the brain by the olfactory nerve, through which the perception of SMELL is transmitted to the brain.

olfactory nerve the nerve that connects the brain with the olfactory bulb in the cranium, and this with the smell sensors of the nose.

oligodendrocyte one of the delicately branched NEUROGLIA that support the nerve cells of the central nervous system.

oligomenorrhea scanty (or infrequent) menstrual flow.

oliguria the excretion of an abnormally small amount of urine. It may be caused by many factors, including shock, dehydration, or a kidney disorder.

omentum a two-layered fold in the peritoneum (the membrane that lines the abdominal cavity) which hangs from the stomach in front of the intestines. It serves to protect the intestines and limit the spread of abdominal infection.

oncology the study of tumors and their treatment.

oophorectomy the surgical removal of an ovary. It is usually performed when the ovary is diseased or contains a large cyst or tumor.

open-heart surgery surgery during which the heart is opened to operate on its valves, vessels or muscle.

ophthalmology the branch of medical science that deals with the eye and its disorders.

ophthalmoscope an instrument for examining the interior of the eye; it is equipped with a light, mirror and lenses. Using it a physician can examine the retina at the back of the eye.

opiate any drug derived from opium. Morphine and heroin are opiates.

opium a powerful and addictive drug made from the juice of unripe opium poppy seedpods.

optic chiasma the CHIASMA where the two optic nerves cross on their way to the brain.

optician a person who makes or sells eyeglasses and other optical instruments. An ophthalmic optician is medically qualified to give an eye examination and prescribe eyeglasses.

oral contraceptive an alternative name for the contraceptive pill, one of the most popular forms of CONTRACEPTION.

orbit the bony socket that surrounds and protects each EYE.

orchitis inflammation of one or both testicles. It may be caused by injury, infection, or as a complication of MUMPS. The symptoms include swelling and pain sometimes accompanied by fever, nausea and vomiting.

organ any individual part of the body that has a special function. Many organs occur in pairs; this means that if one is damaged the other can continue to carry out its functions.

organ of Corti a sense organ located in the INNER EAR, on the inner surface of the COCHLEA. It changes vibrations of sound into nerve impulses for transmission to the hearing center of the brain.

organ transplant the transfer of an organ from one person to another. The main problem is rejection, if the IMMUNE SYSTEM of the receptor's body regards the new organ as "foreign" and sets out to destroy it.

osteopathy

orgasm the pleasurable climax of the sexual act. In men, the penis ejaculates semen; in women, there are powerful contractions of the vagina and womb.

orthodontics the branch of dentistry concerned with the prevention and correction of irregularities in the position of the teeth.

Osler, William (1849–1919) a Canadian physician who became the first to recognize endocarditis and to trace its origin to a bacterium. Among his more than 700 books and articles was *The Principles and Practice of Medicine* (1892).

osmosis the physical principle by which two fluids of different concentrations — one a strong solution, the other a weak — pass through a semipermeable membrane and become mixed: the weaker passes into the stronger. This principle is not only the basis for kidney dialysis machines, but corresponds also to the way the actual kidneys work.

ossification the forming of bone. It occurs naturally during the development of the FETUS and during childhood and adolescence.

osteoarthritis a chronic disease that involves degeneration and disintegration of the tissues at the JOINTS. It most commonly affects the hips, knees and spine, and may be accompanied by pain and swelling. There are many possible causes, including aging.

osteology the study of the structure and function of bones.

osteomalacia a softening of the bone in adults due to inadequate or diminished mineralization. The symptoms are aching and painful bones, weakness and susceptibility to fractures. There are many causes, including renal disease, but probably the most common is a deficiency of VITAMIN D and CALCIUM in the diet. RICKETS is a similar bone disorder in children.

osteomyelitis or osteitis inflammation of the bone and marrow by bacteria that form pus. The symptoms include fever, sweating, inflamed skin and pain in the bone. Treatment is with large doses of antibiotics or, in chronic cases, surgery.

osteopathy a type of ALTERNATIVE MEDICINE concerned with manipulation of the spine in conjunction with diagnostic and therapeutic sessions of traditional medicine.

otitis   inflammation of the outer ear (otitis externa) or middle ear (otitis media). Inflammation of the inner ear is called LABYRINTHITIS (or otitis interna).

otorhinolaryngology   the branch of medicine that deals with disorders of the ear, nose and throat.

otosclerosis   a disease of the MIDDLE EAR that leads to increasing deafness. It involves a thickening and hardening of one of the small bones in the middle ear, which prevents the bone from vibrating and transmitting sound. A rarer form of otosclerosis similarly affects the inner ear.

otoscope   an instrument equipped with a light for examining the ear canal and eardrum.

ovarian cyst   a round, fluid-filled lump that occurs in the ovary. It may grow to a considerable size and cause pain or bleeding such that surgery may be necessary.

ovary   the female reproductive glandular organ, which produces ova from MENARCHE to MENOPAUSE. It also supplies HORMONES that regulate female secondary sexual characteristics, including the menstrual cycle, and is involved in maintaining early stages of pregnancy.

ovulation   the release of an ovum (egg) from an ovary. It occurs midway through a woman's menstrual cycle.

ovum   an egg, released at ovulation from an ovary.

oxygenation (of blood)   occurs in the alveoli of the lungs during breathing.

oxygen therapy   the administration of oxygen to a patient. Such therapy is given to patients who have an inadequate level of oxygen in the blood, as for example in heart failure or pneumonia.

oxyhemoglobin   a compound of HEMOGLOBIN and oxygen, formed in the lungs, which carries oxygen in the blood.

oxytocin   a HORMONE, released by the PITUITARY GLAND, that stimulates contractions of the WOMB during CHILDBIRTH.

P

pacemaker   part of the heart technically called the sinoatrial NODE. Its function is to initiate, maintain and regulate the heart rate by means of regular electrical impulses. An artificial pacemaker (sometimes called cardiac pacemaker) is a temporary or permanent apparatus that is surgically implanted in the body to take over a diseased node's functions.

Paget, James (1814–1899)   a famous nineteenth-century surgeon, physician, and medical teacher in Britain. In 1876 he described a chronic disease of the bones characterized by inflammation and deformation. He called it *osteitis deformans*, later to be renamed Paget's disease.

pain   the sensation of acute mental or physical suffering that results from damage to nerves or innervated body tissues.

painkilling drugs   *see* ANALGESICS.

palate   the roof of the mouth, separating it from the nasal cavity. The hard palate is at the front; the soft palate at the back.

palpation   a medical examination of an area of the body using the hands.

palpitation   abnormally rapid or irregular beating of the heart. It is most commonly caused by deep emotion or sudden shock, but may also be a symptom of heart disease.

palsy   *see* PARALYSIS.

pancreas   the digestive and endocrine organ that secretes enzymes into the adjacent DUODENUM. INSULIN is produced in the endocrine cells of the pancreas, the ISLETS OF LANGERHANS.

pancreatitis   inflammation of the pancreas, commonly caused by GALLSTONES or ALCOHOL abuse. The acute form may be accompanied by severe pain, fever and vomiting. Chronic pancreatitis is marked by pain in the upper abdomen and back, nausea, vomiting and malabsorption.

pannus   a growth of vascular connective tissue on the surface of the synovial membranes of a joint, often seen in rheumatoid ARTHRITIS. Such tissue may also form on the cornea as a complication of the eye-membrane infection trachoma.

Papanicolaou, George

Papanicolaou, George (1883–1962) an American anatomist, born in Greece, who devised the PAP TEST for the early detection of cervical CANCER (now usually called a cervical smear test).

Pap test a test for cancerous development in cells from certain parts of the body, named after George PAPANICOLAOU. It is used most effectively as the smear test for detecting cancer of the cervix.

Paracelsus, Philippus Aureolus (1493–1541), real name Theophrastus Bombastus von Hohenheim a Swiss physician who is regarded as the founder of medical chemistry.

paralysis partial or complete inability to move part of the body. It is usually caused by disease or damage in the nerves that control muscles. One common cause is trauma to the spinal cord. MULTIPLE SCLEROSIS and POLIOMYELITIS also cause paralysis. In a STROKE, the blood supply to a part of the brain is cut off, and the area of the body controlled by that portion of the brain may be paralysed.

paranoia a condition marked by intricate delusions of persecution, which cannot be dispelled even in the face of logic or objective proof.

paraplegia PARALYSIS of the lower limbs. Its many possible causes include damage to the spinal cord.

parasite any animal or plant that lives in or on another (the host) from which it obtains its sustenance.

parasympathetic nervous system part of the AUTONOMIC NERVOUS SYSTEM.

parathormone (PTH) a hormone secreted by the PARATHYROID GLANDS in the neck, which in part regulates the level of CALCIUM in the blood.

parathyroid glands four small oval glands in or behind the thyroid gland in the neck. They secrete PARATHORMONE.

Paré, Ambroise (1510–1590) a French physician who is regarded as the father of modern surgery. He gained valuable experience as an army surgeon, and was the first to use tourniquets in amputations instead of cauterizing the flesh with hot oil.

parietal of the walls of a body cavity, which may be structured of bone (as in the parietal bones of the skull) or of membrane (as in the parietal PLEURA).

Parkinson's disease, or Parkinsonism   a chronic, slowly progressive neurological disease of the middle-aged and elderly. Symptoms include muscular rigidity and tremors that shake the whole body, a set face with unblinking eyes, and a characteristic shuffling gait. Symptoms may be controlled to some extent by medical treatment, but there is no cure.

parotid glands   two glands, located one in front of each ear, part of the salivary apparatus. They release SALIVA into the mouth as food is being eaten or when it is anticipated.

parotitis   inflammation of the parotid glands, as in MUMPS.

parturition   the process of CHILDBIRTH.

Pasteur, Louis (1822–1895)   a French immunologist who was one of the founders of the science of microbiology. The process of PASTEURIZATION, named after him, is a technique used today to destroy harmful microorganisms in food. He made many other valuable contributions to medicine, chemistry and bacteriology.

pasteurization   a method of preparing drinks such as milk or wine, or solid foods such as cheese, by heating to a specific temperature in order to destroy disease-producing bacteria.

patch test   a skin test used to detect and identify a specific ALLERGY. A small sample of the suspected substance is applied to the skin and two days later the skin is examined for signs of allergic response.

paternity test   a test to determine if it would be possible for a particular man to be the father of a specific child. Present techniques are based on an analysis of the BLOOD TYPES of the child and the alleged father, and as a result, can prove only that a man is not the father, or that he may be the father — but not that he is.

pathogen   popularly called a germ, any substance that can cause disease.

pathology   the branch of medicine that studies changes in the body caused by or causing disease.

Pavlov, Ivan (1849–1936)   a Russian physiologist who became famous for his experiments demonstrating the CON-DITIONED REFLEX in dogs. He also carried out valuable researches into the circulation of the blood. In 1904 he was awarded the Nobel Prize for physiology and medicine.

pectoral of or relating to the chest.

pediatrics the branch of medicine concerned with the growth, development and disorders of children.

pediculosis the condition of being infested with any one of various types of LOUSE.

pellagra a disease caused by a lack of NIACIN in the diet. Niacin is part of the VITAMIN B complex. The condition is characterized by itching, scaling of the skin, diarrhea, and a variety of neurological abnormalities.

pelvis the cradle of three pairs of bones — ilium, ischium and pubis — that supports the base of the spine, holds the abdomen and provides the attachment for the bones of the legs. The term is also used for the part of the KIDNEY where the URETER collects urine.

Penfield, Wilder Graves (1891–1976) an American surgeon, professor of neurology and neurosurgery at McGill University. His experiments with epileptic patients to find the source of permanent memory in the brain convinced him that the temporal region was part of an automatic mechanism that scanned the record of the past.

penicillin the original and one of the most valuable antibiotic drugs. It is derived from a compound originally obtained from *Penicillium* molds. It kills bacteria that cause many infections, but has no effect on viruses.

penis the erectile sexual organ in the male; it also contains the URETHRA.

pepsin an enzyme produced in the stomach that breaks down proteins into smaller molecules called peptides, to permit their further digestion.

peptic ulcer an ULCER of the STOMACH or DUODENUM that is thought in some way to be related to the secretion of gastric acids.

perception awareness of what it is that we experience through the senses, such as vision, hearing, the senses of smell and taste, and so on.

percussion a procedure commonly used by physicians to diagnose irregularities, particularly of the lungs. A finger is placed on the relevant part of the body and is tapped by a finger of the other hand. The quality of the sound emitted gives the doctor a clue to the condition of the underlying structure.

pericardium the membranous sac surrounding the HEART.

pericarditis inflammation of the PERICARDIUM.

perineum the skin and fibrous tissues of the body region between the legs, from the anus to the scrotum or vulva.

period a common term for the menstrual period, or the duration in days of MENSTRUATION.

peripheral nervous system the entire nervous system of the body apart from the CENTRAL NERVOUS SYSTEM (the brain and spinal cord).

peristalsis the involuntary muscular contractions that occur in various tubular vessels of the body. In the ESOPHAGUS and INTESTINES it helps to move food along.

peritoneum the membrane that lines the abdominal cavity and covers the INTESTINES, STOMACH, and other abdominal organs.

peritonitis inflammation of the PERITONEUM. It is a potentially dangerous disorder that can result from infection (such as through a ruptured appendix) or irritation.

pernicious anemia a form of ANEMIA which results from an inability by the small intestine to absorb vitamin B_{12}.

personality disorders persistent and maladaptive styles of responding to and interacting with other people and the environment.

perspiration, or sweat a salty fluid secreted through the skin, mainly as a means of cooling the body. It is produced by sweat glands.

pertussis, or whooping cough an acute, highly contagious respiratory infection. It is caused by a bacterium and generally affects children under the age of ten. The early stages resemble a heavy cold with a persistent cough, which increases in violence with the sound of a whoop as the breath is drawn in. A vaccine is available that gives protection from this disease.

Perutz, Max (1914–) an Austrian-born British biochemist who demonstrated the structure of HEMOGLOBIN. His lengthy and painstaking work was recognized by the Nobel Prize in chemistry for 1962.

pessary a suppository (a capsule soluble at body temperature) inserted into the vagina or anus.

petit mal a minor seizure that is accompanied by little or no abnormal movement, and may involve only momentary unconsciousness.

Pett a scanning system in which harmless radioactivity is used to provide a cross-sectional image of the body for diagnostic purposes.

Pfaffman, Carl (1913–) an American electrophysiologist who has pioneered the electrophysiology of taste. His researches into the sensory codes of neural impulses and the gustatory pathways to the brain have contributed much to physiological psychology.

pH a measure of the acidity or alkalinity of a solution. pH values up to 7 are acid; 7 is neutral; above 7 is alkaline. The pH of normal blood is between 7.35 and 7.45.

phagocyte any cell capable of engulfing and destroying foreign bodies, such as bacteria. White BLOOD CELLS which are phagocytes include neutrophils, histiocytes and monocytes.

phalanges the bones of the fingers or toes.

phantom limb the sensation that a limb, or part of it, still exists after it has been amputated.

pharmacology the science or study of DRUGS, including their composition, uses and effects.

pharmacopeia an authoritative listing of medicinal drugs with their composition, usual dosages, effects and other relevant information.

pharyngitis an infection or inflammation of the PHARYNX.

pharynx the area of the throat from the

back of the mouth to the top of the ESO-PHAGUS through which food passes, and the back of the nasal passages to the top of the LARYNX.

phenylketonuria (PKU)   a rare inherited disorder marked, unless treatment is given from birth, by degrees of mental retardation. It is caused by lack of a certain enzyme, producing an accumulation of the AMINO ACID phenylalanine.

phlebitis   inflammation of a VEIN, often associated with THROMBOSIS, which is a blood clot in a blood vessel. The condition may be precipitated by prolonged bed rest, and may thus be considered a complication of surgery.

phlegm   another word for MUCUS or SPUTUM in the respiratory passages.

phobia   an extreme, persistent, and abnormal dread of something, for no apparent reason. It is classified as a type of anxiety disorder.

physiotherapy   the treatment of injuries, physical defects and pain by means of exercise, heat, massage, and other physical methods.

pia mater   the inner of the three MENINGES, the membranes that cover the brain and spinal cord.

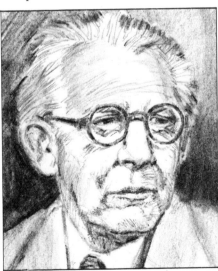

Piaget, Jean (1896–1980)   a Swiss psychologist who spent most of his life studying the reasoning powers of children, and from this contributed significantly to the knowledge of human intellectual development.

pigmentation coloration caused by the presence of pigments, natural substances produced in the body. Rhodopsin (visual purple) in the retina of the eye is essential to vision, red HEMOGLOBIN in the blood carrries oxygen; and the dark pigment MELANIN protects the skin from the harmful effects of ultraviolet radiation.

piles *see* HEMORRHOIDS.

"pill" the popular name for an oral contraceptive, used for CONTRACEPTION.

pimple a small round, inflamed swelling in the skin containing PUS. A rash of pimples is called ACNE.

pineal body a pea-sized gland in the brain, of which the exact function is unknown.

pink eye *see* CONJUNCTIVITIS.

pituitary gland, or hypophysis an outgrowth from the underside of the brain beneath the HYPOTHALAMUS. Hormones from the pituitary regulate the function of many other glands.

PKU *see* PHENYLKETONURIA.

placebo a biochemically inactive substance administered as a medication, of which the therapeutic value lies in its psychological effect on the patient. In clinical trials of drugs, the effects of a new drug are compared with the effects of placebos.

placenta an organ that develops in the womb during pregnancy. Derived in part from the outermost embryonic membrane and in part from the uterine wall, it supplies nutrients to the FETUS and collects waste products from it via the UMBILICAL CORD.

plague a highly infectious bacterial disease that is usually fatal if untreated. Bubonic plague, caused by fleas from infected rats and characterized by gross enlargement of lymph nodes, especially in the armpit and groin, eventually also attacks the lungs. Sputum coughed up by victims contains the plague bacteria — which become airborne and infect other humans, causing pneumonic plague. Pneumonic plague is a more virulent form.

plantar reflex a reflex action of the big toe in response to stroking the outer side of the sole of the foot. The toe should point downward. Lack of response or a upward movement indicates a nervous disorder.

pneumothorax

plantar wart, or verruca   a white, hardened patch of skin that appears on the sole of the foot. It is most commonly caught from walking barefoot in changing-rooms and by the side of indoor public swimming pools.

plaque   a colorless, transparent, hard layer of microorganisms accumulated on the teeth, which if not regularly removed can lead to dental caries (decay) and diseases of the gums.

plasma   the clear fluid content of blood and lymph.

plasmapheresis   a method of taking plasma from the body. A quantity of blood is drawn off and the red blood cells separated from it; what remains is plasma.

plastic surgery   surgery that deals with remodeling, repairing and restoring injured or defective surface features. When this is done to improve the appearance it is called cosmetic surgery. Altering the shape or size of the breasts is known as mammoplasty; plastic surgery of the nose is called rhinoplasty. Plastic surgery is also concerned with skin GRAFTS.

platelet   a small disk-shaped body in blood which in the presence of injury adheres to others to form a clot under which healing can begin.

pleura   a double membrane surrounding the lungs and lining the pleural cavity, which permits the lungs to move relatively freely within the ribcage.

pleurisy   inflammation of the PLEURA. Symptoms are fever, coughing and chest pains.

plexus   a network of blood vessels, nerves, or of the lymphatic system. An example is the solar plexus, the network of sympathetic nerves located in the cavity behind the stomach.

PMS   *see* PREMENSTRUAL SYNDROME.

pneumonia   any infection of the lungs in which gas exchange is disturbed because of pus in the air sacs. It may be caused by bacteria, viruses or chemicals.

pneumothorax   the presence of air in the pleural cavity. The air pressure can cause a lung to collapse. The symptoms are sharp pain and breathlessness.

145

poisoning

poisoning the effect on the body of any chemical substance that can injure or impair function. Nerve poisons, which act on the nervous system and cause convulsions and stupor, include alcohol and chloroform. Irritants burn and cause chemical changes: heavy metals, caustic alkalis, and mineral acids are examples. Some poisonous gases kill by impairing the body's oxygen-transporting mechanism.

poliomyelitis (polio), or infantile paralysis an acute viral infection of the spinal cord that attacks the nerves controlling the muscles. Severe cases may end in paralysis and death. Children are most susceptible, but can be protected by vaccination.

polyp any TUMOR on a stalk. Polyps are commonly found in the nose, colon or womb. Many are completely harmless; troublesome ones can be removed.

polyunsaturated fats molecules consisting of long carbon chains with many double linkages. They are thought to be less harmful as dietary fats than are SATURATED FATS.

polyuria the frequent discharging of large amounts of urine. It is symptomatic of KIDNEY DISEASE or DIABETES.

pons a part of the brainstem.

porphyria a group of HEREDITARY metabolic disorders in which an excess of porphyrins (purple organic pigments which help form HEMOGLOBIN) accumulate in the blood or liver. Crisis periods are commonly precipitated by certain drugs (some barbiturates, for example).

portal vein carries blood from the intestines to the liver.

post mortem, or AUTOPSY the medical examination of a dead body, usually to discover the cause of death.

postnasal drip a discharge from the back of the nose into the back of the throat. It may be caused by a heavy cold or an ALLERGY; medical diagnosis is essential.

Pott, Percival (1714–) an English surgeon who identified the first known carcinogen, thus marking the beginning of modern cancer research. He realized that an accumulation of soot in the skin of the scrotum of chimney sweeps caused cancer.

pregnancy the period from conception

to CHILDBIRTH, when a developing fetus is carried within a mother's womb. The average duration to full term is 280 days, or approximately nine months.

pregnancy test   analysis of a woman's urine or blood to determine if she is pregnant.

premature birth   any birth that takes place between the 28th and 36th week of pregnancy, or involving a baby weighing less than 5½lb.

premedication   a drug or combination of drugs given to patients before a general anesthetic. It sedates the patient.

premenstrual syndrome (PMS)   a condition that affects some women for a few days before MENSTRUATION. Symptoms may include depression, irritability, and headache. It is also called premenstrual tension (PMT).

premolar or bicuspid   one of eight TEETH located in pairs in front of the molars each side of the upper and lower jaws.

prepatellar bursitis   a form of BURSITIS that affects the knee; it is commonly called "housemaid's knee" because it may be precipitated by prolonged kneeling.

presbyopia   a condition of the eyes in which there is difficulty in focusing on close objects. It is caused by a hardening and flattening of the lens, common in the elderly.

prescription   the note a physician writes as an instruction to a druggist to dispense a medication.

presenile dementia   *see* ALZHEIMER'S DISEASE.

presentation   the orientation of a fetus in the womb relative to the birth canal just before CHILDBIRTH. Normal presentation is head first; other presentations, such as breech, placental, or transverse may all complicate delivery, some necessitating surgical intervention.

pressure sore   *see* BEDSORE.

primigravida   a woman pregnant for the first time.

proctology   the branch of medicine that deals with disorders of the rectum and anus.

prodromal

prodromal a term which means "coming before." It describes a symptom of an impending disease or an early symptom of a disease.

progesterone a female sex HORMONE secreted by the corpus luteum in an OVARY and by the placenta. It prepares the uterine wall for implantation, and stimulates breast tissue. Progesterone has been used alone and in combination with ESTROGEN as an oral contraceptive.

prognosis a prediction of the probable course and outcome of an illness, based on knowledge of the usual course of the disorder, combined with an awareness of factors that might influence it, such as the case history, age, sex and general health of the patient.

prolactin a hormone released by the PITUITARY gland in women that stimulates the production of milk in the BREASTS after CHILDBIRTH.

prolapse the downward displacement of an organ from its normal position. The WOMB and the RECTUM are two organs occasionally subject to prolapse, particularly in elderly women.

prophylactic protecting from or preventing disease. As a noun, it describes any agent or procedure for preventing disease, such as a vaccine or immunization. The SHEATH is a prophylactic against almost all sexually-transmitted disease and, by association, is loosely called a "prophylactic."

proprio(re)ceptor a sensory receptor that responds to stimuli which come from within the body itself.

prostate gland a gland in men that lies below the bladder, where the vas deferens, which conveys sperm from the testes, joins the URETHRA, which carries urine from the bladder to the penis. Enlargement of the prostate is common in elderly men.

prostaglandin one of more than a dozen highly active FATTY ACID derivatives that are present in many tissues and organs. They are found in the brain, kidneys, prostate gland and lungs, among other sites. What they do and how they do it is not yet fully understood.

prostatectomy the surgical removal of part or all of the prostate gland, often because an enlarged prostate is constricting the URETHRA and impeding urine flow.

prosthesis   the replacement of a missing part of the body, such as a limb or an eye, by an artificial substitute.

protein   any of a group of complex organic compounds that contain nitrogen, hydrogen and oxygen. Human body proteins are synthesized from amino acids derived from protein in the diet; they function as enzymes, immunoglobulins, hormones, and in many other essential roles.

protozoans   one-celled organisms, of which there are many thousands of different kinds. The parasitic protozoan that most commonly infests the human body is an AMEBA which causes a severe form of DYSENTERY.

pruritis   the medical name for ITCHING.

psoriasis   a disease characterized by red flaky patches on the skin and nails. It may occur anywhere or all over the body; it is sometimes associated with ARTHRITIS. The cause is unknown; ointments, creams and drugs are usually remedial.

psychiatry   the medical specialty concerned with the diagnosis and treatment of MENTAL DISORDERS.

psychoanalysis   a method of PSYCHOTHERAPY originally devised by Sigmund FREUD for the treatment of the neurotic and mentally ill. Based on the assumption that the causes of NEUROSIS lie in the psychological history of the patient, often in early childhood, psychoanalysis seeks to bring these unconscious factors into consciousness, where they can be faced by the patient and overcome.

psychology   the science that deals with the study and understanding of the mind and behavior.

psychosomatic   a term describing physical disorders which result mainly from emotional problems. Psychosomatic disorders may have no diagnosable organic cause, but to the person suffering from them they are nevertheless quite real.

psychosis   any severe mental disturbance of organic or psychological origin in which the patient exhbits gross loss of reality testing.

psychotherapy   a way of treating psychological problems that usually involves verbal interaction of a specific and prescribed order between psychotherapist and patient. PSYCHOANALYSIS is a type of psychotherapy, whereas PSYCHIATRY in the strict sense is not.

psychotropic drugs   DRUGS that affect the mind.

puberty   the stage of human development during which the sex organs mature. This begins in girls at about the age of ten or eleven; in boys at about eleven or twelve. It corresponds with the physical and emotional changes of adolescence.

pubis   the front lower part of either of the hip bones, which form the front arch of the PELVIS.

puerperal fever, or childbed fever   a streptococcal infection of the WOMB. It occurs in a mother usually within ten days of childbirth. Now rare, it can be successfully treated with ANTIBIOTICS.

puerperium   a period of six weeks after childbirth. After this, the physiological changes of pregnancy have regressed.

pulled muscle   a popular term for a muscle that has been slightly damaged by a rupture of its fibers. Trained massage and the application of local heat can help.

pulmonary   of or pertaining to the LUNGS.

pulse   the palpable evidence of the HEARTBEAT as felt in an artery. It is most readily felt in the arteries of the forearm, by the wrist (radial artery). There are also prominent pulses in the forehead (temporal artery), neck (carotid artery) and groin (femoral artery).

pupil   the opening in the iris of the EYE, through which light passes to reach the RETINA.

purpura   discoloration of the skin caused by bleeding under the surface. It may be caused by any condition in which the blood vessels have become fragile, or by a deficiency in the normal blood clotting factors. Treatment depends on the specific cause.

pus   a thick liquid that collects at the site of an infection. It is made up of white blood cells, lymph, and the remains of dead bacteria.

pustule a small, inflamed, pus-filled, raised area like a small BOIL. It is a common symptom of ACNE.

pyelogram an X-ray photograph of the kidneys.

pyelonephritis an inflammation of the KIDNEY and its pelvis, the conical upper portion of the URETER. It may be caused by infection that has backed up from the bladder or been introduced through the bloodstream.

pyemia a condition in which PUS sometimes seeps into and poisons the blood, causing abscesses, violent shivering and high fever. The condition calls for urgent treatment with antibiotics.

pyloric stenosis a narrowing of the pylorus, the valvelike outlet between the stomach and the duodenum. It may be a congenital disorder or result from spasm of the pyloric muscle brought on by a peptic ulcer.

pylorus the short, narrow passage that connects the stomach and the duodenum.

pyridoxine one of the chemicals in the VITAMIN B group which contributes to the formation of proteins inside the body.

Q

quadriplegic a person who suffers from PARALYSIS in all four limbs.

quarantine a period of enforced partial or total isolation of someone after exposure to an infectious disease.

quickening the first signs of movement of an unborn baby (fetus) felt by a pregnant woman.

quinine drug extracted from the bark of the cinchona tree. Formerly widely used to treat or prevent MALARIA, it has now been largely replaced by synthetic antimalarial drugs such as chloroquine.

quinsy an acute throat infection in which an ABSCESS forms in the region of the tonsils. It is often a complication of TONSILLITIS, with pus-forming bacteria present. Treatment is by antibiotics and, if necessary, surgery.

R

rabies, or hydrophobia   a virus infection transmitted to human beings by the SALIVA of an infected mammal, usually through its bite. The rabies virus invades the nervous system. Following a bite from a suspect creature, rapid administration of rabies antiserum is essential to halt the progression of this formerly invariably fatal infection, before the inevitably lethal encephalitis sets in.

radiation sickness   a condition that results from overexposure to high-energy radiation from radioactive sources, such as radium or X rays. Symptoms include vomiting, diarrhea and burns. Eventually there is a loss of hair, impaired gait, anemia, convulsions, infertility and possibly leukemia or other forms of cancer.

radioisotope   another word for a radioactive ISOTOPE, sometimes used in radiology for diagnosis and treatment.

radiology   the study of radiant energy — X rays, GAMMA RAYS and radioactive substances such as RADIOISOTOPES — in the diagnosis and treatment of disease.

radiopaque   describes anything opaque to radiation, especially X rays. Radiologists use radiopaque substances that can be swallowed or injected to visibly distinguish internal parts of the body.

radiotherapy   the treatment of disorders using radiation. For example X rays, radium, and other radioactive substances can be used to destroy unwanted living tissue, such as a TUMOR.

radius   one of the two bones of the forearm, the other being the ulna.

Ramón y Cajal, Santiago (1852–1934)a Spanish physician who became one of the world's leading histologists. An expert microscopist, he became particularly interested in the nerve cell. He was able to prove that the NEURON is the basic unit of the nervous system.

rapid eye movement (REM) rapid movement of a sleeper's eyeballs under closed eyelids while in one of the stages of sleep that coincides with DREAMING.

rash   an area of localized and temporary inflammation of the skin. There are many causes including INFECTION and ALLERGY.

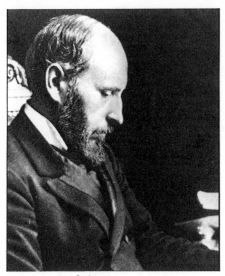

Ramón y Cajal, Santiago

recessive   in genetics, a term applied to genes that are secondary in determining inherited characteristics to the corresponding DOMINANT genes.

rectum   the last part of the INTESTINES, between the COLON and ANUS.

red blood cell, or erythrocyte   the disk-shaped BLOOD CELL containing HEMOGLOBIN that transports oxygen (and carbon dioxide) in the blood.

referred pain   pain that is felt in the body at a location other than the site of the causative disorder. The location of referred pain is usually characteristic, however; for instance, the pain of APPENDICITIS may be felt on the left but not the right side of the lower abdomen.

reflex, or reflex action   an automatic involuntary muscular response to a stimulus. A typical example is the KNEE JERK. One type of psychological reflex is called a CONDITIONED REFLEX.

reflex arc   a short nerve pathway between a point of stimulation and the responding muscle or gland, by-passing the brain. Many involuntary automatic responses depend on this arc.

regurgitation   the surging back of fluid or food into the mouth or esophagus from the stomach. It differs from vomiting in that it is not associated with nausea, nor is it accompanied by abdominal muscular contractions.

relapse the return of symptoms of a disorder after an apparent recovery.

REM *see* RAPID EYE MOVEMENT.

remission an interval within the course of a chronic illness during which the patient's symptoms decrease or even disappear. Remission may be the result of therapy, or it may be spontaneous.

renal insufficiency the reduced capacity of the KIDNEYS to function normally.

renin an ENZYME produced by the KIDNEYS; its principal effect is to raise the blood pressure.

replacement surgery, or spare-part surgery surgery intended to replace damaged or absent parts of the body with natural or synthetic substitutes. It contrasts with TRANSPLANT SURGERY, which involves replacement with donated living tissues.

respiration the process of breathing in and out. Oxygen, taken in from the air to fill the lungs, is carried in the bloodstream to the tissues of the body. There it is consumed as it provides energy for the cells. The resulting waste products include CARBON DIOXIDE. This is released into the lungs and expelled into the air when a person breathes out.

respiratory center the regulator of breathing in the MEDULLA OBLONGATA, part of the BRAINSTEM.

resuscitation the use of any one of several methods to restore breathing (and heart action) to someone in whom one or both have ceased. Resuscitation of breathing is called ARTIFICIAL RESPIRATION; combined with heart massage to restart a stopped heart it is called CARDIOPULMONARY RESUSCITATION.

retardation usually refers to MENTAL RETARDATION.

reticular activating system a system of brain cells consisting of the reticular formation together with the pathways that run up to it along the SPINAL CORD. It contributes to the physical basis of consciousness.

retina the tissue of light-sensitive cells that line the back of the EYE.

rhesus factor (Rh factor) an inherited substance in the BLOOD of most people, who are classified as Rh positive. If the factor is absent, they are Rh negative.

rheumatic fever a disorder that follows a streptococcal infection of the throat which has been left untreated. It involves inflamed joints, fever and a rash. Sometimes it may also lead to permanent damage of the heart valves (VALVULAR DISEASE OF THE HEART). More common in children and adolescents, rheumatic fever is thought to be an AUTOIMMUNE DISEASE induced by ANTIGENS to the streptococcus bacteria.

rheumatism a general term used to describe pain and stiffness in the joints and muscles.

rheumatoid arthritis chronic inflammation of the joints, which become stiff and swollen and are eventually deformed. The cause is not known, and treatment is usually restricted to painkilling drugs.

Rh factor incompatibility *see* HEMOLYTIC DISEASE OF THE NEWBORN.

rhinoplasty PLASTIC SURGERY on the nose, usually carried out for cosmetic reasons.

riboflavin a VITAMIN in the vitamin B group that infuses energy and promotes general health; it is a constituent in many foods.

ribs twelve pairs of curved, flattened bones that surround and protect the chest cavity.

rickets a form of OSTEOMALACIA in children that results from a deficiency of VITAMIN D. The bones are thus prevented from properly absorbing calcium and phosphate and, as a result, become soft and malformed. Children with rickets are restless and pale, and may suffer from seizures.

ringworm (medical name, tinea) a contagious fungus infection of the skin, despite its name. The affected area becomes inflamed and spongy, and eventually peels and flakes. Damp, warm places of the body are usual sites for ringworm, especially between the toes. There, the condition is more usually known as ATHLETE'S FOOT.

rods the light-sensitive cells in the RETINA which respond best to low-intensity light. Unlike CONES, they do not distinguish color.

Rogers, Carl (1902–) an American psychologist who founded humanistic psychology. Rogers's innovative therapeutic approach discarded the conventional teacher-pupil relationship and instead allowed patients to decide how progress was to be made, in a friendly person-to-person relationship.

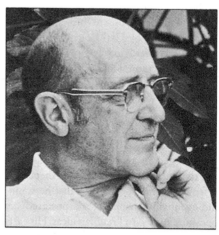

Rorschach test *see* INKBLOT TEST.

rosacea (acne rosacea) a skin complaint that results from a malfunction of the SEBACEOUS GLANDS in the skin. It usually affects the face.

roseola (roseola infantum) thought to be a virus infection; it affects only young children. Symptoms include a high fever followed by a pink rash.

rubella, or German measles a contagious virus disease that shows itself as a pink rash. Although the symptoms are mild, the disease can be dangerous to an unborn child if contracted by the mother in the first trimester of pregnancy; it may result in congenital abnormalities such as heart defects, mental retardation and deafness.

rubeola *see* MEASLES.

rupture the common name for a HERNIA.

S

sacroiliac joint the joint formed by the meeting of the SACRUM and the pelvis bones at the base of the spine.

sacrum a bony triangle made up of five fused bones just above the coccyx, at the base of the SPINE.

"safe period" the time during a woman's menstrual cycle when sexual intercourse is calculated not to lead to conception. Intercourse is avoided for about three days before and two days after OVULATION.

saliva a slightly alkaline mixture of watery MUCUS secreted by the salivary glands into the mouth. Its function is to moisten the mouth, soften the food, permit taste and commence digestion of carbohydrates.

Salk, Jonas Edward (1914–) an American medical researcher who in 1952 developed the first successful vaccine to immunize against polio (POLIOMYELITIS). Salk selected three strains of the virus, and killed them to make a vaccine.

Salmonella a genus of rod-shaped bacteria that sometimes cause food-poisoning. *Salmonella typhi* is the cause of typhoid fever.

salpingitis inflammation of a Fallopian tube, or less commonly, of a Eustachian tube.

Sanger, Margaret (1883–1966) an American pioneer of birth control. She trained as a nurse and, after witnessing the fatal effects of an illegal abortion, devoted the rest of her life to bringing CONTRACEPTION information to all women. She was the founder and first president of the American Birth Control League, and in 1922 toured the world on behalf of the movement.

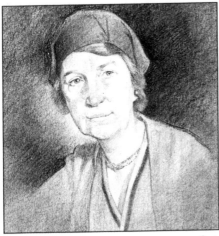

sarcoma any cancerous TUMOR that forms in connective tissue, including the muscles or bones.

saturated fats FATS which, because of the arrangement of their carbon and hydrogen atoms, cannot absorb additional hydrogen. Most animal fats are saturated, and many experts believe that an excess of them in the diet has a causative effect in such disorders as ARTERIOSCLEROSIS.

scabies a contagious skin infection caused by the itch mite. It burrows into the skin and lays its eggs there, causing itching and redness.

scanning a modern diagnostic procedure that uses computer-enhanced radiography or sonography to create "pictures" of a patient's interior, generally on a video screen.

scapula the anatomical name for the shoulder blade.

scar (medical name, cicatrix) a mark left on the skin after the healing of a sore, injury, burn or cut. Small scars usually fade away in time. Large scars may be effaced or improved by PLASTIC SURGERY.

scar tissue tough, fibrous tissue that forms a SCAR. A KELOID scar is characterized by unusual thickening of the tissue.

scarlet fever, or scarlatina a streptococcal bacterial infection that mainly affects children. Symptoms include sore throat, fever and vomiting. Later, a rash of tiny red spots appears over the body. The disease is now swiftly and successfully treated with antibiotics.

schizoid a personality characterized by emotional coldness and indifference to the feelings of others, with few or no close relationships.

schizophrenia, formerly called dementia praecox any of a group of serious mental disorders of greater than six months' duration marked at some point by bizarre delusions or auditory hallucinations. There is inevitable deterioration from previous levels of functioning in work and social life.

Schwann, Theodor (1810−1882) a German naturalist who is widely regarded as being the founder of cell theory. Schwann also discovered pepsin, and studied the laws of muscular contraction and of fermentation and putrefaction.

sciatica severe pain along the sciatic nerve which runs from the lower back into the legs. It may often be a referred symptom of a SLIPPED DISK.

sclerosis the hardening of tissues or organs because of the growth of fibrous tissue within them or the accretion of material upon them.

scoliosis sideways curvature of the spine. It may result if one leg is shorter than the other, or it may be produced by poor posture. More serious causes include hip and spine diseases.

screening the testing of a large number of people who are apparently well for the presence of disorders by using only the basic part of the usual examining processes.

scrofula the former name for TUBERCULOSIS of the LYMPH NODES. Young children are the main victims, but the disease is now rare.

scrotum the skin-covered sac containing the TESTES, which lies outside the male body behind the PENIS.

scurvy a disease caused by a lack of VITAMIN C (ascorbic acid). Symptoms are fatigue, weakness, bleeding gums and lowered resistance to infection. Scurvy can be prevented by a balanced diet, especially one containing fresh fruit.

sea sickness a type of TRAVEL SICKNESS caused by the pitching or rolling of a boat.

sebaceous cyst a CYST that is formed from an oil-secreting gland in the skin.

seborrhea a mild disorder of the sebaceous glands in the skin. It is characterized by excessive secretion of sebum, the glands' natural oil. Layers of dead cells eventually start to flake off the skin (as dandruff, in the scalp).

sebum a natural oil secreted by the sebaceous glands in the skin. It helps to protect against bacteria and serves as a lubricant for skin and hair.

secretion the process by which various body substances are released by the cells of glandular organs. The term also describes the substance secreted, such as SALIVA.

sedation the administration of a drug or drugs to calm and soothe an excited patient; also the state of calm that then ensues.

sedimentation rate the rate at which solid elements separate from suspension in a liquid. The term usually applies to the ERYTHROCYTE SEDIMENTATION RATE.

seizure

seizure another name for a CONVULSION.

semen the thick whitish fluid that contains the male sex cells (sperm). It is emitted from the penis during EJACULATION.

semicircular canals the three curved tubelike structures set in three different planes that constitute the organ of BALANCE in the EAR.

seminiferous tubules long, narrow, coiled tubes in the TESTES whose function is to manufacture SPERM.

senility appreciable physical and/or mental deterioration that affects some elderly people.

sensitization the process of becoming immunologically reactive to some specific substance, such as dust or pollen, which occurs in an ALLERGY.

septicemia another word for toxemia or BLOOD POISONING.

septum a dividing partition between two parts of an organ or cavity.

serum the clear, yellowish, watery part of blood that remains after the CLOTTING components and cells are removed.

sex either of two divisions, male and female, into which organisms are classified according to their reproductive functions.

sex hormones chemical controllers of reproduction released by the sex glands in a male (testes) and those in a female (ovaries). They are themselves under the control of master hormones secreted by the PITUITARY GLAND. A male's sex hormones are called androgens; a female's hormones are estrogens and progesterone.

sexual intercourse, or coitus the act of sexual union between a man and a woman.

sexually-transmitted diseases (STD) disorders and infections carried from person to person by sexual contact. They were formerly called venereal diseases (VD). The principal diseases are AIDS, chancroid, gonorrhea, syphilis, and genital herpes.

sheath a device placed over the PENIS to trap sperm and prevent it entering the female partner's vagina during sexual intercourse. It is a common form of CONTRACEPTION.

Sherrington, Charles Scott (1861–1952) an English neurophysiologist who presented the first full, experimentally documented explanation of how the nervous system produces coordinated movements.

shinbone the bone at the front of the lower leg; the common word for the TIBIA.

shingles an infection caused by the virus HERPES zoster. It inhabits the nervous system and produces pain and blisters in the skin. The same virus causes CHICKENPOX.

shock a set of symptoms brought on by a sudden deep emotional disturbance or by sudden physical injury. Emotional shock can occur alone, or it can be associated with physical, or "organic" shock, which is the more dangerous of the two. Physical shock is marked by loss of blood pressure, cold sweat and difficulty in breathing.

shortsightedness (medical name, myopia) a common eye defect which can be corrected with eyeglasses or contact lenses. It occurs because the image is focused in front of the retina, not on it.

shoulder blade the common name for the SCAPULA.

Siamese twins, or conjoined twins identical twins who at birth are joined together, most commonly at the chest, shoulder, hip, or head. They are sometimes successfully separated surgically.

sickle-cell anemia a hereditary chronic form of anemia almost exclusively confined to black people. Deoxygenated red blood cells become sickle- or crescent-shaped; as a result, the cells cannot easily pass through the capillaries, leading to possible thrombosis.

side effects undesirable secondary effects resulting from a drug or other form of medical treatment.

SIDS (sudden infant death syndrome), also called crib death a mysterious disease, believed to be respiratory, that kills babies in their cribs. There are usually no warning symptoms.

silicosis an OCCUPATIONAL DISORDER of the lungs caused by breathing silica (quartz) dust over a period of years.

Sims, J. Marion an American physician who became a pioneer of gynecological surgery. In 1855 he established in New

York the first hospital for women in the United States.

sinus   an enclosed space or cavity, often filled with blood or air. The term is commonly applied to the air-filled cavities in the bones of the skull near the nose.

skeletal muscle, or striated muscle   one of the names for the striped voluntary MUSCLE tissue that is under the control of the MOTOR CORTEX in the brain.

skeleton   the body's bony framework.

skin   the outer covering of the body, made up of two layers, the EPIDERMIS and the DERMIS.

skin graft   a transplant or GRAFT of skin tissue from one part of a person's body to another where the skin has been destroyed, often as a result of a BURN.

Skinner, Burrhus Frederic (1904 –   )
an American psychologist who established BEHAVIORISM as a legitimate branch of psychology.

skull, or cranium   a bony container made up of twenty-two bones that houses the brain and the organs of balance, sight, hearing, smell, and taste.

sleep   a periodic state of unconsciousness from which it is comparatively easy to emerge. Sleep seems to be essential to the central nervous system for rest and recuperation, and for the general physical health of the body.

sleeping pills   DRUGS taken to induce a state of sleep.

sleepwalking (medical name, somnambulism)   a sleep disorder characterized by walking about and performing various actions while fast asleep, eyes shut *or* open. After waking, the person usually remembers nothing of what has occurred.

slipped disk (medical name, herniated intervertebral disk)   a condition that results when one of the rings of cartilage between the vertebrae of the spine becomes displaced and compresses the spinal cord or a nerve.

smallpox   a highly contagious viral infection. The most virulent form was generally fatal, but following a worldwide program of IMMUNIZATION, the disease has been eradicated.

smear test   another name for the CERVICAL SMEAR TEST or PAP TEST.

smell, sense of   detects chemicals that dissolve in the fluids covering the olfactory membranes of the nose. This stimulates the olfactory nerve which conveys the "message" to the brain.

Smith, Hamilton Othanel (1931–   ) an American molecular biologist who isolated a bacterial enzyme that cut DNA at specific sites, and who was the first to identify the gene fragments thus produced. He shared the 1978 Nobel Prize in physiology and medicine with Daniel NATHANS.

smoking   the deliberate inhalation of the fumes from burning substances, most commonly tobacco. It can lead to a physical and psychological addiction that damages health. Cigarette smoking in particular damages the lungs, blood vessels, heart and many other organs,

smooth muscle   involuntary MUSCLE under the control of the AUTONOMIC NERVOUS SYSTEM and, in certain cases, the ENDOCRINE SYSTEM. Most of the internal organs of the body contain smooth muscle.

snakebite   an injury that requires emergency treatment to counteract the effects of the poison. If the snake is identified, the specific ANTIVENIN should be injected into a muscle or a vein.

sneezing   a violent, involuntary expulsion of breath from the nose and the mouth caused by irritation inside the nose. It may be the result of infection, inflammation, or an ALLERGY, or the inhalation of some irritant such as dust.

snoring   noisy breathing during sleep. It is caused by the vibration of the soft PALATE, located at the back of the roof of the mouth.

Snow, John (1813–1858)   an English physician who administered chloroform to Queen Victoria at the birth of Prince Leopold in 1853, and by doing so ensured public acceptance of ANESTHESIA for pain relief in childbirth. He also proved that CHOLERA is transmitted by contaminated water.

solar plexus   the nerve PLEXUS behind the stomach, consisting of ganglia of the SYMPATHETIC NERVOUS SYSTEM innervating abdominal organs.

SKIN

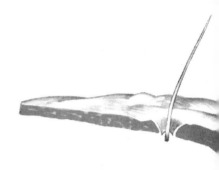

Skin is made up of a series of layers. On the surface is a layer of dead cells. A fraction of an inch below this is the living epidermis. Here skin cells are constantly renewing themselves.

Below the epidermis is the thicker dermis. Within it are glands that secrete oil or seb[um] to lubricate and waterproof t[he] skin, and sweat glands, whos[e] actions help maintain a constant body temperature. Hairs grow in follicles within the dermis. Nerves and bloo[d] vessels are also found in the dermis.

The skin's color is determined by the activity of cells in the epidermis called melanocytes. The melanocytes produce the pigment melanin, and the darker the skin the more melanin they make. Melanin production is also stimulated when the skin is exposed to sunlight and produces a sun tan.

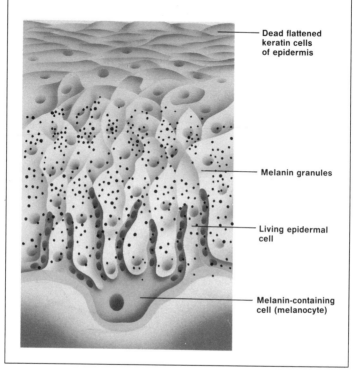

Dead flattened keratin cells of epidermis

Melanin granules

Living epidermal cell

Melanin-containing cell (melanocyte)

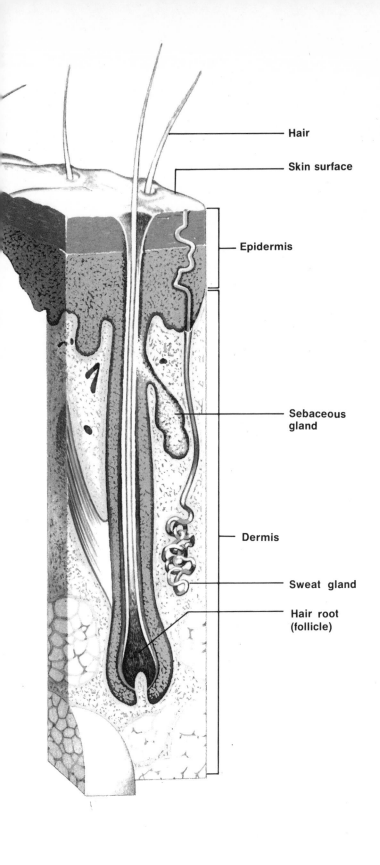

Hair

Skin surface

Epidermis

Sebaceous
gland

Dermis

Sweat gland

Hair root
(follicle)

somnambulism the medical name for SLEEPWALKING.

sonography a technique that uses high-frequency sound waves (ultrasound) for diagnostic purposes. Tissues reflect ultrasound waves, creating echoes which are detected by a receiver and processed by a computer to create a visual image.

spare-part surgery *see* REPLACEMENT SURGERY.

spasm the sudden involuntary contraction of a muscle, usually accompanied by pain.

spastic produced by spasms, involuntary muscular contraction. Spastic paralysis, for example, is an inability to voluntarily move a limb in which the muscles are constantly tensed.

spectacles *see* EYEGLASSES.

speech the faculty of speaking — making intelligible and meaningful sounds that are generated by the VOCAL CORDS and GLOTTIS in the LARYNX and modified by the mouth, tongue, palate, lips and teeth.

speech therapy treatment for speech disorders and defects.

Spemann, Hans (1869–1941) a German embryologist who pioneered research into the mechanics of embryological development. He was awarded the Nobel Prize in physiology and medicine in 1935.

sperm, or spermatozoon the male generative cell, produced in the testes. The word sperm is also used to refer to the SEMEN ejaculated, which contains millions of spermatozoa.

spermicide substance that kills SPERM. It is used as a form of CONTRACEPTIVE.

Sperry, Roger (1913–) an American psychobiologist whose research into the mysteries of "split-brain" patients earned him the Nobel Prize in medicine in 1981. He discovered that the CORPUS CALLOSUM, a major neural pathway of the brain, serves as a link between the two cerebral hemispheres.

sphincter a ring of muscle surrounding the opening of a hollow organ or body. When it contracts it partly or completely closes the opening.

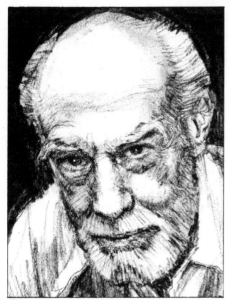

Sperry, Roger

sphygmomanometer an instrument used to measure BLOOD PRESSURE.

spina bifida a birth defect affecting the covering of the spinal cord. The bones of the spine are not properly joined and fail to afford protection for the spinal cord. Some kinds of spina bifida are associated with paralysis.

spinal cord the extension of the CENTRAL NERVOUS SYSTEM from the brain, which is contained within and protected by the vertebral column.

spinal nerves the thirty-one pairs of nerves that branch out from the SPINAL CORD to various parts of the body. They carry impulses to and from the central nervous system and themselves form the major part of the peripheral nervous system.

spinal puncture another name for LUMBAR PUNCTURE.

spine, or spinal column the chain of VERTEBRAE from the base of the cranium to the tip of the coccyx. It consists of seven cervical, twelve thoracic, five lumbar, five sacral and four coccygeal vertebrae.

spirochete a spiral-shaped order of BACTERIA.

spleen an organ located behind the stomach just below the diaphragm. Its primary functions are to remove damaged red blood cells from the circulation, to store reserve PLATELETS, and to elaborate LYMPHOCYTES.

splint any device or appliance used to support an injured part of the body by keeping it rigid and preventing its movement.

Spock, Benjamin (1903 –) an American pediatrician whose original book, *Baby and Child Care* (1946), had a tremendous influence on child care throughout much of the Western world.

spondylosis OSTEOARTHRITIS of the SPINE. The joints of the spine are narrowed as the disks that separate the vertebrae degenerate. Spondylosis does not always produce symptoms, but when present they may include stiffness in the neck, and pain and numbness in an arm or hand.

sprain damage to a joint in which the ligaments are overstretched. Pain and swelling accompany the condition.

sprue a disorder of the digestive system in which there is failure by the small intestine to absorb fat and vitamins properly.

sputum, or phlegm matter, largely MUCUS, that is coughed up from the lungs and windpipe into the mouth.

squamous cell a flattened epithelial cell.

squint (medical name, strabismus) a condition in which the alignment of the eyes is not parallel. It is usually caused by weakness in the muscles of one eye.

stammering, or stuttering a speech defect marked by involuntary hesitation and repetitions, usually of the first syllable of a word.

stapes a tiny bone in the MIDDLE EAR. Shaped like a stirrup, it conducts sound by vibrating the oval window of the inner ear.

staphylococcus a type of spherical BACTERIUM.

starch a common type of CARBOHYDRATE, found particularly in potatoes, wheat, rice and corn.

Starling, Ernest Henry (1866 –1927) an English physiologist who was the first to define a HORMONE — a substance produced by one tissue which had an effect on another tissue.

stenosis abnormal narrowing of a tube or duct in the body, either by accretion of material within the tube, or by thickening of the tube wall.

sterility the inability to produce off-spring. The term also means a state of being germ-free.

sterilization conferring STERILITY. In the context of CONTRACEPTION, however, it refers to a surgical process in which the TESTES or OVARIES are removed, or the routes (VAS DEFERENS or FALLOPIAN TUBE) by which germ cells (SPERM or OVA) travel from them are blocked.

sternum the breastbone, to which the ribs are attached at the front of the chest.

steroid one of a group of DRUGS and chemicals which have effects similar to those of the steroids produced by the ADRENAL GLANDS (CORTICOSTEROIDS).

stethoscope an instrument used by physicians to listen to sounds within the body (for example, the heartbeat). It consists of a hollow disk which amplifies sound through a tube connected to earpieces.

stillbirth the birth of a fetus that has died in or after the 28th week after conception. Occurring before that, the death and natural expulsion from the womb of a fetus is called a miscarriage.

stimulants DRUGS that have a stimulating effect on any body activity.

stitches a common term for SUTURES.

stomach the large muscular organ in the alimentary canal at the top of the abdomen that begins the major breakdown of foods in the digestive process.

stomach pump a suction pump attached to a flexible tube which is inserted into the patient's mouth or nose and down the esophagus into the stomach to empty part or all of the contents.

stone a common term for a CALCULUS.

stool another word for FECES.

strabismus *see* SQUINT.

strain in a physical sense, an injury to muscle through overuse, marked by pain around the area and stiffness. It differs from SPRAIN, which is generally more serious. Emotionally, strain is a mental tension of which the symptoms may include irritability and insomnia. Mental strain is similar to STRESS.

streptococcus a genus of BACTERIA responsible for many infections and diseases.

stress mental or physical reaction to some overpowering external stimulus. Emotional stress may follow events that cause fear, worry, or depression. Localized physical stress may result from repeated impact on any part of the body.

striated muscle *see* SKELETAL MUSCLE.

stroke, cerebrovascular accident, or apoplexy a sudden loss of consciousness, or paralysis, resulting from a blocked or ruptured blood vessel in the brain causing damage to brain tissue.

stroke volume the amount of blood pumped out by the left VENTRICLE of the heart at each beat into the aorta.

stuttering *see* STAMMERING.

stye a boil on the eyelid caused by the bacterial infection of a gland on or under the eyelid.

styptic any substance that prevents bleeding by causing local blood vessels to contract. Alcohol, alum and silver nitrate may be used for this purpose.

subconscious the mental stratum that lies below the level of normal consciousness. No longer in common use, the term denotes both the preconscious, which can be recalled with effort, and the unconscious.

subcutaneous just under the skin.

sudden infant death syndrome, or crib death *see* SIDS.

sulfa drugs sulfonamide DRUGS, which prevent or inhibit bacterial growth.

sunburn, or suntan the result of prolonged exposure to the sun's rays. Suntanning of light-skinned people by the sun's ultraviolet rays can be achieved with moderate exposure; over-exposure can result in HEATSTROKE and second-degree BURNS.

sunstroke *see* HEATSTROKE.

superego in PSYCHOANALYSIS, the element of personality concerned with ethics, morality and social self-consciousness, in contrast to the instinctive ID and the mediating EGO.

suppuration   the process by which the body forms and discharges PUS.

suprarenal gland   another name for the ADRENAL GLAND.

surgery   the branch of medicine that treats injuries and diseases by means of internal manipulation or operation. It is usually associated with incision into the body by a specialist.

surrogate   a substitute, or a replacement.

suture   the stitching together of two bodily surfaces; commonly, the stitches which repair a wound or a surgical incision. In anatomy, a suture is the fused junction between bones, such as those of the SKULL.

swallowing   the process of passing food and other substances from the mouth to the throat, down the esophagus toward the stomach. During swallowing, a flap of cartilage called the epiglottis seals off the breathing passages (larynx and trachea), thus stopping food and drink from entering the windpipe.

sweat   the salty fluid secreted from the sweat glands in the skin, in the process of sweating or PERSPIRATION to cool the body.

sympathetic nervous system   part of the AUTONOMIC NERVOUS SYSTEM. It prepares the body for emergency action by speeding up the heartbeat, dilating the pupils, and relaxing the bladder, among other functions.

symptom   any abnormality in the function, feeling or appearance of the whole or part of the body that indicates the presence of disease.

synapse   a tiny gap marking the junction between two nerves.

syncope   the medical term for FAINTING.

syndrome   the collection of signs and symptoms that together constitute the clinical presentation of a specific disease or disorder.

synovial fluid   a clear lubricating fluid secreted by synovial membranes, the connective tissue lining the joints. The membranes can become inflamed (*see* BURSITIS).

syphilis, or lues   a SEXUALLY-TRANS-MITTED DISEASE caused by a spiral-shaped bacterium. The primary phase starts as a sore on the genitals, anus or lips. The second stage is marked by generalized illness and debility, and a rash of highly infectious ulcers.

syringe an instrument used for injecting fluid into or drawing fluid from the body. A HYPODERMIC syringe has a tube fitted with a fine nozzle and a plunger. A hollow needle is fitted to the nozzle.

systole the contraction of the VENTRICLES of the heart, when the cardiac muscles squeeze blood from the ventricles into the aorta.

T

tachycardia an abnormally fast heartbeat.

talus the bone of the ankle, with which the TIBIA and FIBULA of the lower leg articulate.

tampon a plug of absorbent material inserted into a body cavity or open wound in order to absorb secretions or stop the flow of blood. The term commonly describes a menstrual tampon which is inserted into the VAGINA to absorb fluids produced during MENSTRUATION.

tapeworm a parasitic worm which attaches to the inside of the intestines. Typically a tapeworm has a long, segmented ribbon-like body. Special drugs can rid a patient of the infestation.

tarsal any one of the seven bones of the INSTEP of the foot.

taste the sense perceived when the taste buds of the TONGUE are stimulated. These detect sweet, salt, sour and bitter tastes.

Tatum, Edward Lawrie (1909 –1975) an American biochemist who is regarded as the founder of biochemical GENETICS. He shared the 1958 Nobel Prize in physiology and medicine for his part in the discovery that each gene is responsible for one specific enzyme, thus contributing to the overall regulation of biochemical processes.

Taussig, Helen (1898 –   ) an American physician who was instrumental in the development of an operation to save "blue babies" by establishing a surgical procedure to increase blood flow to the lungs. This was first used successfully on babies in 1944.

TB *see* TUBERCULOSIS.

tears the watery, salty secretions of the LACRIMAL GLANDS of the EYE.

teeth bonelike structures set in the jaws for biting and chewing. A full adult set totals thirty-two teeth made up of eight incisors, four canines, eight premolars, and twelve molars. Each has a root, or roots, a central pulp cavity filled with blood vessels and nerve endings, a thick layer of generative DENTIN and a hard protective cap of ENAMEL. The teeth are fixed by their roots in the bones of the jaw (MAXILLA or MANDIBLE), and are surrounded by the fleshy GUMS.

teething the process by which a baby's teeth first grow through the gums.

temperature a measurement of heat. An adult's normal body temperature, taken with a thermometer under the tongue, is about 98.6°F (37°C).

tendon the tough band of tissue that connects MUSCLES to the parts of the body on which they act, usually to bones.

tennis elbow a painful condition of the elbow caused either by a strain of the ligaments of the forearm, or by BURSITIS of the elbow joint.

tension a state of being stretched; it is also another word for STRESS which increasingly denotes emotional tension.

teratogen any agent that causes malformation or other abnormalities in a developing EMBRYO, which is particularly vulnerable in the first three months of pregnancy.

testis, or testicle male sex gland, equivalent to the female OVARY. It is the site of sperm manufacture in an adult, and produces most of the male sex HORMONES.

test meal RADIOPAQUE food or drink given to a patient before being X-rayed to examine the condition of the esophagus, stomach, or intestines. The most common type is a BARIUM MEAL.

testosterone a male sex HORMONE produced mainly by the testicles. It promotes the physical changes in adolescent boys that make them sexually mature. In females (produced by the adrenal glands) testosterone controls the distribution of body hair.

test-tube baby a baby that has developed from an egg fertilized in vitro, then introduced to the mother's womb in the hope that it will implant in the lining.

tetanus, or lockjaw a disease characterized by painful muscular spasms caused by the toxin of the bacterium *Clostridium tetani* which lives in the soil. Wounds coming into contact with contaminated soil may permit the bacteria to enter the body. Vaccination can be used to prevent or treat tetanus.

thalamus a region of the brain concerned with the reception of sensory information. It connects with the HYPOTHALAMUS and with the CEREBRAL CORTEX.

thalassemia a type of inherited anemia which involves an abnormal breakdown of the red blood cells. In its severe form it is often fatal before the age of thirty.

thermometer an instrument for measuring temperature. Two types of clinical thermometers are used: one (oral) placed under the tongue; the other (rectal) inserted into the rectum. Oral thermometers are also used to record the axillary temperature in the armpit.

thiamine *see* VITAMIN B₁.

thirst a feeling of dryness in the mouth and throat coupled with a desire to drink. Abnormal thirst may be a symptom of illness.

thorax the part of the body known also as the chest or ribcage between the neck and the abdomen. It contains the lungs and heart, and is bordered by the diaphragm, ribs, thoracic vertebrae and clavicles. Major vessels within the thorax include the trachea (windpipe) and esophagus (gullet), and the vena cavae, aorta and other blood vessels to and from the heart.

thrombosis the formation of a blood clot in a blood vessel, thus obstructing the flow. In an artery, thrombosis can lead to an infarct, gangrene or a stroke. In the coronary arteries, a thrombosis causes a HEART ATTACK.

thrush (medical names, candidiasis, moniliasis) a fungal infection that may appear in the mouth, vagina, or anywhere moist and warm. The term thrush is most commonly used when this disease affects the throat, however. Thrush is infectious and grows often when the body's immunity to it has been weakened by drugs, hormone imbalance, or some other condition.

thumb the first and sturdiest of the five digits of the hand. Unlike the other digits, it has only two bones, not three.

thymus a gland of lymphatic tissue concerned with the IMMUNE RESPONSE in babies, children and adolescents. It is located in the thorax above and in front of the heart. After PUBERTY it tends to shrink.

thyroid gland an endocrine gland located in the neck in front of the windpipe, that secretes important hormones into the bloodstream.

thyroxine a hormone secreted by the THYROID GLAND, concerned with the regulation of metabolism. A shortage of thyroxine causes HYPOTHYROIDISM.

tibia the shinbone, the larger of the two bones of the lower leg.

tic an involuntary twitching, usually of the face, head, neck or shoulders.

tic douloureux *see* TRIGEMINAL NEURALGIA.

tinea a general name for fungus diseases of the skin, particularly RINGWORM.

tinnitus ringing, buzzing, or other noises in the ear. It may be the result of a build-up of wax in the ear, or it may be a symptom of disease (such as MENIÈRE'S DISEASE or OTITIS), but in many cases the cause is not known.

tissue a group of cells of the same general type, which have their own function in the body.

toe one of the five digits of the foot.

tolerance the body's capacity to endure the effects of pain or of a drug or poison. Tolerance to DRUGS can be built up by taking progressively larger doses of a substance over a prolonged period. This may be an aspect of ADDICTION.

tomography one of several techniques for taking X-ray pictures of "layers" of the human body at selected angles. This is effected by moving the X-ray camera around the patient, who remains stationary. In conjunction with a computer, this process can present full cross-sections of the patient on a video screen (a CAT scan).

tongue a flat, muscular organ in the mouth that serves as the principal organ of TASTE. It is also important in chewing and swallowing, and in SPEECH.

tonsils paired masses of lymphatic tissue located at the back of the throat. They are valuable in helping to combat invasion of the body by harmful bacteria.

tonsillitis inflammation of the TONSILS, which may be caused by either a bacterium or a virus. Antibiotics can now usually clear the infection, making unnecessary the previously common surgical removal of the tonsils (tonsillectomy).

tooth *see* TEETH.

toothache pain most commonly caused by decay (dental caries) that has penetrated the two outer layers of a tooth, the enamel and dentine, and reached the nerves in the pulp of the tooth.

tooth decay (medical name, dental caries) the progressive breakdown of the enamel, dentin and root of one or more TEETH by bacterial action. Erosion of the enamel begins with the formation of PLAQUE on the tooth.

torticollis *see* WRYNECK.

touch, sense of a reaction to pressure on the skin by bulblike nerve endings called touch receptors located in the skin.

tourniquet a tightening device applied above a wound in a limb to stop the blood flow. A tourniquet should be applied only by professional medical staff.

toxemia, loosely called BLOOD POISONING the presence of bacterial toxins in the blood.

toxemia of pregnancy a potentially life-threatening condition that occasionally affects women in their first pregnancy. The symptoms include swelling of the limbs and face, and high blood pressure. Untreated it may develop into ECLAMPSIA, a highly dangerous condition.

toxin is any poisonous substance produced by a living organism. Bacteria can form various kinds of toxins. Toxoids, derived from them, may be used as VAC-CINE.

trace elements elements that are needed in minute amounts in order to maintain essential body processes. Common trace elements include aluminum, copper, fluorine and silicon.

trachea, or windpipe the cartilaginous tube through which air passes between the nasopharynx and the bronchi of the lungs. It includes the LARYNX.

tracheostomy a surgical operation in the throat to create an opening in the front of the TRACHEA (windpipe).

traction a steady pull on a limb that contains a fractured bone once it has been reset correctly, in order to hold the parts in the correct end-to-end position as they heal. It is also used to treat spinal nerve compression.

trance a sleeplike state, as in deep HYPNOSIS and some aspects of HYSTERIA.

tranquilizers drugs that reduce nervous tension.

transfusion an injection or infusion of fluids (usually blood, plasma or saline). A blood transfusion is a means of supplying a patient with blood that is not his or her own. The blood, of the correct BLOOD GROUP, may come from a single donor, or be prepared as a blend by a blood bank.

transplant surgery the replacing of diseased or damaged parts of the body with healthy parts. A part to be transplanted may be taken from a live donor or from one who has just died, or from elsewhere in the patient. The rate of success depends on preventing the body from rejecting the replaced part.

transvestism the urge that derives sexual pleasure from wearing clothes of a person of the opposite sex.

trauma medically, any physical injury or wound. Psychologically, the term describes a powerful mental shock which may eventually lead to NEUROSIS.

travel sickness, or motion sickness a sense of NAUSEA, sometimes accompanied by VOMITING, that is felt by some people when traveling in a moving vehicle. It is primarily caused by movement of the fluid in the SEMICIRCULAR CANALS of the ear.

TONGUE

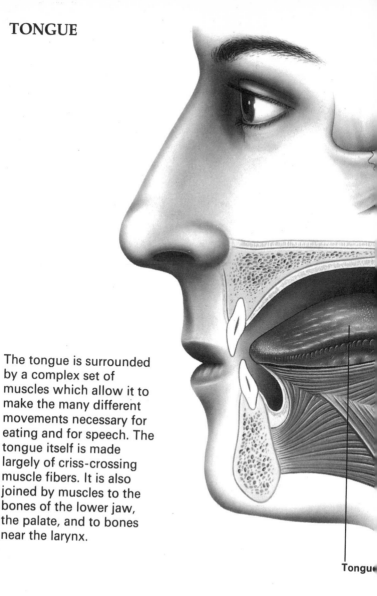

The tongue is surrounded by a complex set of muscles which allow it to make the many different movements necessary for eating and for speech. The tongue itself is made largely of criss-crossing muscle fibers. It is also joined by muscles to the bones of the lower jaw, the palate, and to bones near the larynx.

Tongue

The taste buds of the tongue are grouped in different ways according to the taste sensations they detect. Sweet tastes are discerned by buds at the tip of the tongue, sour and salt ones at the sides, and bitter ones at the back. The overall sensation experienced when food is eaten is a mixture of these four basic tastes.

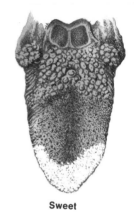

Sweet

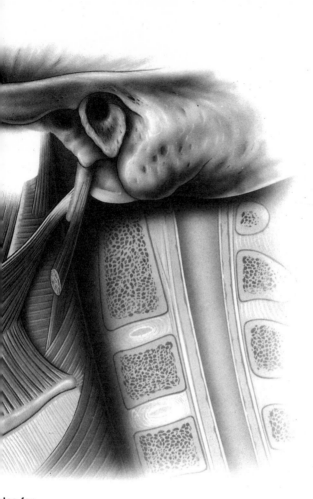

les for
e movement

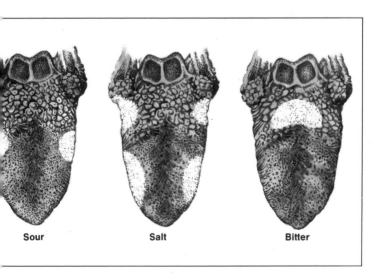

Sour   **Salt**   **Bitter**

tremor   an involuntary trembling in the muscles. Mental factors such as excitement or anxiety may produce tremors. Physical causes include nervous disorders, disease of the liver or kidneys, or MULTIPLE SCLEROSIS. A tremor may also be a symptom of a disorder, for example PARKINSON'S DISEASE, or may result from SENILITY or ALCOHOLISM.

trephination   a surgical operation that involves removing circular sections of bone from the skull.

trigeminal neuralgia, or tic douloureux   a sudden sharp pain on one side of the face, caused by an acute disorder of the trigeminal nerve. This is the complex, branched nerve that transmits information between the face and the brain. The condition more commonly affects the elderly.

trisomy 21   another name for the genetic disorder DOWN'S SYNDROME.

tuberculosis (TB)   an infectious disease caused by a bacterium. It usually affects the lungs but it may also attack the intestines, kidneys, nervous system, larynx, bones or skin. Most commonly caught by breathing in the germs, tuberculosis is generally treated with antibiotics over a long period.

tumor   an abnormal growth of tissue. BENIGN tumors do not spread elsewhere in the body. MALIGNANT tumors (CANCER) are made up of cells that do multiply and spread.

tunnel vision   a condition in which the eyes seem to focus only on what is being looked at directly; the rest of the visual field is severely blurred. Causes are various, including the onset of MIGRAINE or advanced chronic GLAUCOMA.

twins   two children born of the same mother at the same time. Non-identical or fraternal twins, who may be of different sexes, develop from two different eggs that were fertilized at the same time. Identical twins, who are always of the same sex, develop from a single fertilized egg that subsequently splits in two.

tympanum, or tympanic membrane   the medical name for the EARDRUM.

typhoid fever   a bacterial infection acquired by eating food or drinking water that has been contaminated by the excreta of infected persons. Symptoms are high fever, abdominal pain and slow pulse. Treatment is with antibiotics.

typhus   a group of highly contagious diseases caused by microorganisms called Rickettsiae and carried by fleas, ticks and mites. The symptoms of all forms include high fever and a rash of pink spots on most parts of the body. Treatment is with antibiotics.

U

ulcer   an inflamed open sore in the skin or in a mucous membrane. Among the many types of ulcers are gastric or peptic, in the stomach; and duodenal, in the duodenum.

ulcerative colitis   inflammation and ulceration of the colon. Bloodstained diarrhea is a major symptom, accompanied by fever and abdominal pain. Chronic ulcerative colitis may eventually lead to cancer of the colon.

ulna   one of the two bones of the forearm, the other being the RADIUS.

ultrasound   vibration or oscillation of a frequency above the audible range. It is used in SONOGRAPHY as a diagnostic aid.

ultraviolet radiation   electromagnetic radiation in the range of wavelengths just beyond the violet end of the visible spectrum. Such rays cause suntan and produce VITAMIN D in the skin; excessive quantities damage or destroy living tissue, however.

umbilical cord   a long, flexible tube that links a FETUS with the PLACENTA in the mother's WOMB. Its function is to supply food and oxygen to the fetus and to facilitate the discharge of waste products.

umbilicus   the medical name for the navel, the scar in the center of the abdomen where the umbilical cord was attached before birth.

unconsciousness   the state of being insensible. The condition may vary from stupor (semiconsciousness) to COMA.

undescended testicle   *see* CRYPTORCHIDISM.

urea   a chemical formed in the LIVER from ammonia derived from proteins. It is found in the blood, urine and lymph.

ureter   the tube between the funnel-like pelvis of the KIDNEY and the BLADDER.

urethra   the tube that carries URINE away from the bladder. In males it extends through the PENIS and also carries semen.

urethritis   inflammation of the URETHRA. It may be caused by ordinary local infection or by SEXUALLY-TRANSMITTED DISEASE. Symptoms are a painful discharge and frequent urination.

uric acid   one of the body's waste products excreted in the URINE.

urinary tract   the passage and all the organs associated with the making and discharge of URINE. Urine is produced in the KIDNEYS. From there it flows down two URETERS and into the BLADDER. It is discharged from the bladder through a tube called the URETHRA.

urine   the watery solution of waste products removed by the KIDNEYS from blood, and excreted through the URINARY TRACT. Analysis of the chemical composition of urine is a valuable diagnostic aid, particularly for disorders such as DIABETES and NEPHRITIS, and certain heart, metabolic and liver disorders.

urology   the branch of surgery concerned with diseases and disorders of the URINARY TRACT.

urticaria   *see* HIVES.

uterus   *see* WOMB.

uvula   a small fleshy flap of tissue that hangs from the soft palate at the back of the mouth. It has no known function.

V

vaccination   a technique for conferring immunity against specific diseases that consists of injecting a VACCINE into the body.

vaccine   a preparation containing germs or their products which is injected into the body. It may consist of dead germs; live but weakened germs, which multiply harmlessly in the body; or a toxoid, which is a harmless form of the disease being treated. Immunity arises as a result of the ANTIBODIES formed naturally following this injection.

vagina   the muscular passage of the

female reproductive tract between the WOMB and the VULVA.

vaginitis inflammation of the VAGINA. It may be caused by a fungus, protozoan, or bacterial infection.

vagus nerve the tenth CRANIAL NERVE and the main nerve of the PARASYMPATHETIC NERVOUS SYSTEM.

valve a fold or flap of tissue inside or at the edge of a tubular structure or cavity in the body, shaped so that fluids can pass in one direction easily but will close the valve if they try to flow the other way. Valves occur in the veins of the legs, to help the flow of blood back to the heart. The most important valves in the body, however, are in the heart itself, between the atria and ventricles and between the ventricles and the aorta and pulmonary arteries.

valvular disease of the heart a group of disorders that affect one or more of the four valves of the heart. The condition may be congenital, or RHEUMATIC FEVER can cause scarring and other damage to the valves.

varicella *see* CHICKENPOX.

varicose vein a vein that has become distended and twisted because of the high pressure of blood passing through it. Such veins may occur in any part of the body, but the superficial veins of the lower legs are most commonly involved.

variola *see* SMALLPOX.

vas deferens the tube that carries SPERM from the testicles into the ejaculatory duct via the prostate gland and seminal vesicles.

vasectomy male STERILIZATION by removing part of the VAS DEFERENS. This stops sperm from reaching the penis but does not affect sexual performance or experience, and so is an effective form of CONTRACEPTION.

vasoconstriction narrowing of the caliber of the blood vessels, caused by constriction of the smooth muscle within the walls of the blood vessel. Vasoconstriction is a normal response of blood vessels in the skin when exposed to cold; it also occurs when EPINEPHRINE or NOREPINEPHRINE is released in anticipation of danger or urgent activity.

vasodilation, or vasodilatation widening of the walls of the blood vessels through the action of the muscles within them. It occurs when the body is warm and needs to cool the blood by letting it flow near the surface of the skin; it can also be stimulated by DRUGS, of which alcohol is a common example.

vector, or carrier an agent that transmits a disease without suffering the symptoms. Mosquitoes are vectors of MALARIA; rats and rat fleas are vectors of PLAGUE.

vein a vessel that carries deoxygenated blood from the tissues back toward the heart.

vena cava either of two major veins that empty blood into the right atrium of the heart. The superior vena cava carries blood from the head, neck and arms; the inferior vena cava returns blood from the chest, abdomen and legs.

venereal diseases see SEXUALLY-TRANS-MITTED DISEASES.

venom any poisonous fluid that can be injected into the body through a bite or sting from an insect, a reptile, or another creature.

ventral the front or anterior surface of the body, as opposed to the DORSAL or posterior surface.

ventricle a small cavity in the body. The term usually refers to the two ventricles of the HEART. The brain also has ventricles, filled with CEREBROSPINAL FLUID.

ventricular fibrillation FIBRILLATION of the VENTRICLES of the heart.

ventricular flutter an extremely rapid beating, called FLUTTER, of the ventricles of the heart.

verruca another name for a PLANTAR WART.

vertebra one of thirty-three bones that together make up the SPINE. The spinal cord runs through a canal penetrating many of these.

vertebral column see SPINE.

vertigo, sometimes wrongly called dizziness a disorder of the balance mechanism. The condition may be a symptom of infection of the middle ear, a reduction of blood flow to the brain, high blood pressure or hardening of the arteries. Drugs — including alcohol — can also produce the effect, which is of being whirled around on the spot at high speed (even if lying down).

Vesalius, Andreas (1514–1564)   a Belgian physician who has been called the father of modern anatomy. He learned his early anatomy by dissecting the corpses of criminals. His great masterpiece, *De humani corporis fabrica* ("On the Structure of the Human Body"), published in 1543, was the standard work on anatomy for more than 200 years.

vesicle   a blister on the skin, such as occurs in chickenpox, or a sac or bladder containing fluid. The seminal vesicles are small sacs containing SEMEN located near the base of the BLADDER and which discharge into the URETHRA during EJACULATION.

villus   a microscopic fingerlike or hairlike projection from the surface of a membrane. The small intestine is lined with villi, which enormously increase its surface area, and therefore its absorptive capacity. The CHORION around an embryo develops villi that attach to the endometrium and ultimately form the PLACENTA.

virulent   highly poisonous; applied to a disease it means having a rapid course and violent symptoms.

virus   a minute organism consisting of a core of DNA and RNA and a protein coat. Viruses are so small they can be seen only with an electron microscope. All are parasitic and can replicate only within a living host cell, using the cell's metabolism.

viscera   the contents of the abdomen.

vision   the normally stereoscopic experience of sight through the EYES.

vitamin   one of a group of chemical substances that are essential, in small quantities, for the proper working of the body. Most are obtained from food. Water-soluble vitamins are those belonging to the B complex and vitamin C. Fat soluble vitamins are vitamins A, D, E, and K. Functions of vitamins are complex and interrelated. In general terms, however, vitamin A is necessary for the proper functioning of the red cells in the retina and for the health of epithelial tissues; vitamin B complex vitamins are necessary for growth, digestion, metabolism, and red blood cell formation; vitamin C is essential for maintaining the structure of cell walls, especially in connective tissue; vitamin D is necessary for calcium and phosphorus metabolism; vitamin E has a general metabolic role, but seems particularly important in maintaining red blood cells and in certain reproductive functions; and vitamin K is important in blood coagulation and clotting.

vitamin deficiency can result from a poorly balanced diet. This in turn may lead to certain deficiency diseases such as SCURVY, RICKETS, and PELLAGRA.

vitreous humor a jelly-like substance that fills part of the eye between the retina and the lens. Like the aqueous humor on the other side of the lens, it is transparent.

vocal cord one of two bands of tissue fixed to the wall of the larynx. Air from the lungs forced between them causes them to vibrate and produce sounds.

voice the sound produced by the vocal cords. The sound is modified by the position of the tongue, lips, palate, cheeks and jaws, and the resonance of the mouth.

vomiting (medical name, emesis) the involuntary ejection of the contents of the stomach through the mouth. This usually happens through a series of muscular contractions that are a reversal of the normal muscular contractions of the stomach.

vulva the opening of the female reproductive tract. It has two pairs of lips (labia): labia majora, the outer and larger pair; and labia minora, the inner pair.

vulvitis inflammation of the vulva. Itching and soreness may stem from an infection such as CANDIDIASIS.

W

wart a skin growth caused by a virus. Warts can be removed by cauterization, but sometimes they disappear without treatment.

Wassermann test a diagnostic blood test for SYPHILIS.

wasting known medically as ATROPHY.

Watson, James Dewey (1928–) an American biologist who in 1962 shared with Francis CRICK and Maurice WILKINS the Nobel Prize in physiology and medicine for working out the molecular structure of DNA (deoxyribonucleic acid).

wax (medical name, cerumen) a fatty substance produced by glands in the outer ear canal. Its function is to trap dust and dirt and so prevent them from reaching the eardrum.

weal a swollen red mark on the skin.

weaning for a baby, substituting a FOR-MULA feed (by bottle) for mother's breast milk, or gradually introducing solid foods.

weight of a person may give a clue to health. Someone who is overweight may be overeating or may be suffering from a glandular disease. A loss of weight without a change of diet or exercise level is also usually an indication of a disorder.

whiplash injury a neck injury caused by a sudden jerk forward of the body such that the head is thrown backward. It is a common injury in car accidents.

white blood cell, or leukocyte any of several types of BLOOD CELL that in general are larger than red blood cells and have nuclei.

whitlow (medical name, paronychia) a small painful inflammation at the edge or base of a fingernail.

whooping cough the descriptive name for PERTUSSIS.

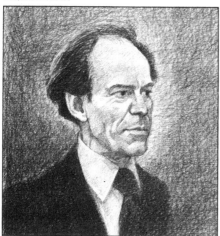

Wiesel, Torsten a Harvard neurobiologist who, with colleague David HUBEL at Harvard, was jointly awarded the Nobel Prize in physiology and medicine in 1981 for research into the nature of VISION.

Wilkins, Maurice Hugh Frederick

Wilkins, Maurice Hugh Frederick (1916–) a New Zealand biophysicist who in 1962 was jointly awarded the Nobel Prize in physiology and medicine with Francis CRICK and James WATSON for his work on the structure of DNA (deoxyribonucleic acid). Using X-ray diffraction techniques, it was Wilkins' discovery of the double helix shape of the DNA molecule that enabled Crick and Watson to determine its molecular structure.

wind a common name for gas or FLATULENCE.

windpipe *see* TRACHEA.

wisdom teeth the molar teeth at the back of the upper and lower jaws. They are the last teeth to erupt, and sometimes erupt crookedly, in which case they may need to be removed.

withdrawal the period that a person suffering an addiction to a drug, such as alcohol or heroin, goes through immediately after the termination of the use of the drug.

withdrawal method, or coitus interruptus a method of CONTRACEPTION in which the male during sexual intercourse withdraws his penis from his partner's vagina before EJACULATION. The probability of some sperm entering the vagina nevertheless is quite high: up to forty per cent.

womb, or uterus the female reproductive organ in which a fetus develops during PREGNANCY. It is normally about the size and shape of a pear. The narrow end, the CERVIX, opens into the VAGINA. Each of two ducts, the FALLOPIAN TUBES, connects the upper end of the womb with an OVARY. The womb itself consists of muscular layers, the innermost of which has a lining (endometrium) that thickens and engorges with blood regularly during the MENSTRUAL CYCLE.

worms primitive animals which — in contrast to bacteria and viruses — have excretory, nervous and reproductive systems. Worms that parasitize humans include FLUKES, roundworms, and TAPEWORMS.

worry a common name for ANXIETY.

wound a break in the skin or internal tissues. It may result from injury in an accident, or from personal violence. The term is also used for the inevitable damage to tissues that occurs during surgery.

wrist the joint between the bones of the forearm and the hand.

wrist drop a condition in which the wrist remains flexed and cannot be extended. The cause is paralysis of the muscles of the forearm.

wryneck (medical name, torticollis) a twisted neck, as may result from injury or muscle spasm. Treatment usually consists of heat, relaxant drugs and physiotherapy.

X

X-chromosome a sex CHROMOSOME. A female has two X-chromosomes; a male has one X- and one Y-CHROMOSOME.

xenophobia a term used in psychiatry to mean a dread of strangers.

xeroderma a skin disorder characterized by rough, dry scales. It is caused by diminished secretions from the glands of the skin, and is usually treated with a prescribed cream.

xerophthalmia, or xeroma a condition marked by abnormal dryness of the CORNEA and CONJUNCTIVA of the EYE. It is caused by vitamin A deficiency, and may be associated with night blindness.

X ray electromagnetic radiation of very short wavelength. The ability of X rays to penetrate soft tissue makes them valuable in diagnosis and in the treatment of diseases such as CANCER, the science called RADIOLOGY.

Y

Yannas, Ioannis an American physical chemist at the Massachusetts Institute of Technology who, in collaboration with John F. Burke, developed a synthetic skin for use with victims of severe burns. It is as thin as a paper towel and biodegradable.

yawning an involuntary action in which the mouth is opened wide after a long breath of air is deeply taken in. It is usually a sign of tiredness or boredom.

yaws a crippling and disfiguring infectious tropical disease. It is caused by a spiral-shaped bacterium and spread by direct contact from person to person through a break in the skin. The symptoms are skin sores that ulcerate and then heal, but five years later — if left untreated — destructive lesions in leg and facial bones occur. Treatment is initially penicillin; if the lesions do occur, surgery is necessary.

Y-chromosome a sex CHROMOSOME. A male has one Y-chromosome and one X-CHROMOSOME. A female has no Y-chromosome, instead she has two X-chromosomes.

yeast a type of one-celled fungus. One variety is used for brewing, and another for leavening bread. A few cause bodily disorders (such as THRUSH).

yellow fever a virus disease carried by the bite of an infected mosquito. The disease attacks the liver, digestive system and kidneys. Malfunction of the liver causes yellow bile pigments to accumulate in the blood, which color the skin. The disease usually involves severe fever, with vomiting and hemorrhaging. Patients require hsopitalization; no cure is known. Preventive vaccination is effective.

yoga a Hindu system of philosophy allied to a course of interrelated exercises and postures designed to promote physical and spiritual well-being.

Z

zinc a mineral that has value to the human body as a TRACE ELEMENT. Zinc oxide, acetate or chloride have antiseptic properties when used externally.

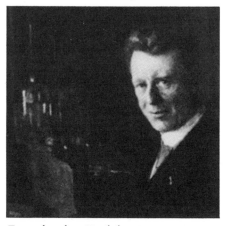

Zwaardemaker, Hendrik

Zwaardemaker, Hendrik (1857–) a Dutch physiologist who specialized in the study of odors. He discovered that the nose adapts to certain odors, and also that two similar odors, inhaled simultaneously will sometimes cancel each other out.

zygomatic arch, or zygoma the slender bony arch on each side of the skull that forms a bridge between the cheekbone and the temporal bone.

zygote a fertilized OVUM.

ILLUSTRATION CREDITS

Photographs

Profession T Blundell, Science Photo Library
Dr Lloyd M Beidler, Biological Sciences, Florida State
University
Ann Ronan Picture Library
Wellcome Institute for the History of Medicine
The Mansell Collection
Dr Brian Eyden, Science Photo Library
Mary Evans Picture Library
Thomas B Allen
Victoria & Albert Museum, Crown copyright
Yale University Library
Thomas B Allen
John Topham Picture Library
Thomas B Allen
Thomas B Allen
Mary Evans Picture Library
Nobelstiften, Sweden
Popperfoto
John T Wood
Thomas B Allen
Thomas B Allen
Wellcome Institute Library, London

Artwork by

Norman Barber
John Bavosi
Louis Bory Associates
Michael Courtney
Mick Gillah
Aziz Kahn
Les Smith
Modern Artz